LIFE AND MORALITY

CONTEMPORARY MEDICO-MORAL ISSUES

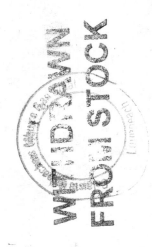

LIFE AND MORALITY

CONTEMPORARY MEDICO-MORAL ISSUES

DAVID SMITH

Gill & Macmillan

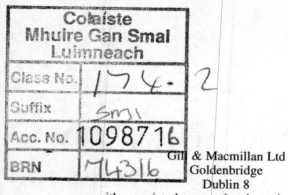
Gill & Macmillan Ltd
Goldenbridge
Dublin 8
with associated companies throughout the world
© David Smith 1996
0 7171 2172 0

Index compiled by Helen Litton
Print origination by *Deirdre's Desktop*
Printed by ColourBooks Ltd, Dublin

1 3 5 4 2

CONTENTS

CONTENTS

INTRODUCTION

This century has experienced both the heights of human scientific ingenuity and the depths of human depravity. Many of these scientific breakthroughs have been of enormous benefit to humanity. To take a few examples: the development of the technology of flight has ensured that our world has shrunk. People now contemplate a journey of thousands of miles without a second thought. Mass communications and the mass media guarantee that events are relayed to us as they occur; the Gulf War aptly illustrates this point. In the comfort of our living rooms we were able to watch the unfolding of the scud missile attack on Tel Aviv. Not only does the mass media ensure that we are 'informed' about wars and catastrophes, but it also endeavours to keep us abreast of new scientific developments and the possible benefits and dangers which these advances might bring.

In the field of medical science some truly remarkable achievements have been realised. Diseases which were once killers are now either completely eradicated or controllable with the use of drugs. Heart by-pass operations, kidney and liver transplants and the like are now common practice in our highly technical hospitals. These medical strides have benefited vast numbers of people and guaranteed them a better quality of life. Rather than focus on a wide range of medical procedures and the ethical questions which can arise I intend to concentrate on only four: abortion; in vitro fertilisation; genetics and euthanasia. This does not mean that other fields of medical science and practice, such as psychology, psychiatry etc., do not also pose important ethical questions. However, the four areas addressed have entered into everyday debate and continue to cause intense controversy within all sections of human society.

Abortion, as we are all aware, is neither a new medical procedure nor a new moral issue. From time immemorial people have resorted to different techniques and drugs to ensure that unwanted pregnancies were terminated. However, the twentieth century has been marked by an 'acceptance' of and legislation for abortion within most cultures, no matter what their philosophical or religious foundations. There are many reasons for this development, some of which will be discussed later. However, there seems to have been a fundamental recognition by legislators that because of the diverse convictions that are maintained on this issue within society the common good demands that abortion should not only be permitted but also controlled by the state and medical profession. Condemnation and support for this interpretation of the common good can be found in most moral traditions. Even though abortion is legal in many jurisdictions and acceptable, under certain circumstances, to some religious traditions, abortion still remains an issue for many people.

The birth of Louise Brown in 1978 as a result of the in vitro fertilisation technique was of significant scientific and social importance. Now for the first time the prospect of remedying certain types of infertility became a real possibility. However, this procedure and the accompanying manipulation of the embryo raised important moral considerations. Questions regarding the moral status of the embryo, parenthood, surrogacy, embryo experimentation and storage of spare embryos now had to be addressed. Equally important was the concern of what these procedures were doing to the women themselves and what they were saying about women in general. Would they transform the way that men view women, or would they usher in new forms of male domination? The media frequently reports new 'advancements' in this field, such as older women giving birth. Once again a debate on the morality of this procedure is generated. What is apparent is that moral theology is having to confront dilemmas which it had never previously encountered, thus necessitating a process of continual reflection and reappraisal.

The relatively new science of genetics has raised considerable expectations and hopes. In the foreseeable future genetically inherited diseases will be able to be diagnosed at a very early stage, and treated. It is hoped that hereditary diseases will be eradicated from afflicted families. But there are also serious apprehensions as well. Will these discoveries ultimately benefit humanity or could they lead to new forms of discrimination and possible abuse?

The question of euthanasia and assisted suicide has now entered the common domain and has become a notable topic of discussion. Certain countries such as the Netherlands and the Northern Territory of Australia permit its practice, while in the United States and in some European countries there is a growing demand for legislation to permit its application in some form. The reason for this increased interest, in the developed world, is probably due to a rapidly ageing population and to the advanced medical procedures which are now currently available. Many commentators believe that in the next decade the central debate will focus on the degree to which society will permit euthanasia and assisted suicide.

Any investigation of these topics immediately unearths a diversity of views on the morality involved in their practice. This is also evident within the different Christian denominations. If individual Christian denominations act as if they have a monopoly on the truth, particularly in these specific areas, they fail to confront a common question well summarised by David Sheppard, the Anglican Bishop of Liverpool: how to react to other Christian traditions who in conscience disagree about particular conclusions.[1] A number of reactions are possible to this diversity within Christianity. Traditionally the inclination has been to disregard convictions which deviated from one's own. Blame for this diversity is attributed to either a lack of mature judgment or an inability to respond to divine revelation as manifest in the Scriptures and in the community. Responses like this have led to a deepening of the divides within Christianity. Another approach, however, is possible. If in attempting to understand the sincere convictions of other denominations we are embarking more fully on the common search for truth, within the framework of the whole Christian tradition we will be better equipped to respond to the new moral dilemmas with which medical science continues to confront us.

Daily life involves decision-making. In the specific domain of the commencement and ending of life people are often called upon to make difficult and traumatic decisions. Many couples have to decide whether or not to keep a pregnancy or abort it. Others decide to embark upon a lengthy, intrusive, and often costly in vitro procedure so that a child may be born. Others have to decide whether or not to be genetically tested to verify whether they are carriers of an hereditary, debilitating disease which could be passed on to their progeny. When faced with the prospect of a terminal illness, patients have to decide whether or not to accept the treatment offered and the implications this will have for their quality of life and for their families. What is abundantly clear is that exacting decision-making is part of human life. But what processes do people employ to facilitate appropriate decision-making? People are inclined to consult authoritative figures or groups within their society to assist them in this process. Traditionally, religious leaders held a position of authority within society. However, today, for a variety of reasons, there has been a gradual decline in the teaching authority of religious leaders. People tend now to consult a variety of authorities to assist them in their decision-making. No prime position is given to any particular authority. They are no longer satisfied to listen to and then act on the pronouncements of their respective churches. Rather, it is becoming increasingly evident that people now aspire to have some personal input into their decision-making. Decision-making, therefore, is made within the context of interlocking relationships and no longer relies on the application of abstract formulations.

This process can be understood as an acceptance of the right to self-determination. Obviously the interpretation of this right is varied and limited. But it appears that an increasing number of people are coming to accept it as the basic premise within which they make decisions which affect their own lives and the lives of their families and society. People now believe that it is their right to determine who they should marry and for how long that marriage will last. They also recognise that it is their right to determine the number of children they will have and the spacing of the birth of each child. Some people go so far as to argue that they have a right to determine the sex and other physical and mental attributes of their children. People also argue that they have a right to abort a pregnancy within certain conditions. Similarly they believe that they have a right to know about their genetic make-up and what effect this will have on their lives and on the lives of their offspring. People have also come to accept that they have a right to choose when they should end their lives. We see a recognition of this right in civil jurisdictions with the decriminalisation of suicide and attempted suicide. Now there is a movement to extend this right to include assisted suicide and euthanasia.

The reasons for the emergence and dominance of the right to self-determination are complex. It could be argued that an interweaving of educational systems, urbanisation, the mass media and individualism are important factors. Whatever the reasons, the right to self-determination is an issue which needs to be recognised by theologians. Theology, if it is to impact on people's lives, must recognise the context within which it operates. For the moral theologian the present context is a pluralistic world in which people assert the conviction that they have a right to determine their lives. This means that moral theology has to find a new role for itself. No longer can it construct essentialist precepts and then strive to implement them in all situations and circumstances. Moral theology should be engaged in the process of facilitating people to make informed moral decisions. In the post-Second Vatican Council era moral theology moved from a manualist approach to an ideal-centred approach. The basic inspiration of this approach still remains valid; but now it has to ensure that the ideal is firmly rooted within the context of people's lives. Rather than furnishing ready-made answers to dilemmas it must ensure that people are equipped to theologise within the context of their lives. A theology which strives to fulfil this methodology will not only address the process of decision-making, but hopefully will ensure that people arrive at mature Christian decisions.

This publication is an attempt to recognise the context in which people find themselves. It endeavours to furnish the relevant data on four significant moral issues, probing the ethical concerns raised and how different Christian denominations have responded to them. Essentially it is intended to facilitate the reader to respond to the new moral dilemmas which currently occur in daily life and in medical practice.

1

ABORTION: A MORAL CONTROVERSY

CONTEXTUAL EVIDENCE FOR THE OCCURRENCE OF ABORTION

Abortion,[1] which is defined as 'an untimely delivery voluntarily occurred with intent to destroy the fetus',[2] is now legal, with varying restrictions, in large parts of the world. Various studies point to an annual abortion rate of forty to fifty million, one for every 2.8 live births. Some countries have a staggeringly high rate of abortion. Recently the *Moscow Business Times* reported that 95% of Russian women had between eight to twenty abortions during their fertile lives.[3]

Any study which attempts to address the practice of abortion in human society cannot avoid enquiring, however briefly, into why women resort to abortion and which socio-economic groups they represent.

Political and economic systems, despite disparate cultures, are the central reasons for many people in many parts of the world today not wanting as many children as their ancestors did. Among the numerous reasons for this shift in attitude are the advances in industrialisation and technology, with accompanying social, cultural, economic and often political changes; as well as increasing urbanisation, invariably a concomitant of industrialisation. Other reasons include an improvement in medicine and public health, which have drastically cut infant mortality rates; and finally, in some areas, a food shortage caused by excessive population growth and a world economic system based on capitalist principles. When these factors converge the ideal appears to be smaller families. These are amongst the arguments vigorously advocated by international agencies such as the *Family Planning Federation* and various United Nations agencies dealing with contraception and population control. Therefore, where contraceptives are non-existent or ineffective, abortions are resorted to as a means of fertility control. Even where abortions are illegal they are still resorted to, often at great risk to the health of women. Rumania is a good example of this. During the dictatorship of Nicolae Ceaucescu abortions were declared illegal. In the following years a slight increase in the birth rate was noted, but a dramatic increase in the mortality rate of women was also observed; this was principally due to women resorting to illegal abortions which were conducted by unqualified persons in unhygienic circumstances.

Another factor which has occurred within recent years is the advance in medical technology, particularly in the diagnosis of fetuses which are either physically or mentally disabled. Increasing numbers of couples are deciding, for a variety of reasons, that they are unable to parent a disabled child and therefore resort to termination of the pregnancy. These diagnostic techniques can also be used to determine the sex of the fetus. In cultures where sons have a higher value than daughters, if these techniques are used and a female fetus is identified, there can be family, social and economic pressures applied to abort her.

In short, analysis suggests that the induced-abortion rate is correlated with urbanisation, socio-economic status, parity and marital status, but relatively independent of religion or cultural background.

Duration and gestation

Nearly all women who want an abortion seek advice before the twelfth week of pregnancy. Mild degrees of legal reform, a cautious medical profession, and in particular, decision-making committees are associated with a high proportion of abortions spilling over into the second trimester. Sweden, with its committee system, is a prime example. In Japan, by contrast, readily available services and a straightforward law permits more than 95% of women to obtain terminations at 12 weeks or less. Young, unmarried mothers are an exception to the generalisation that delay in abortion often depends on the provider. These girls can be slow to recognise pregnancy, and often delay talking to their parents or seeking help; and in this respect, as in many others, they present particular problems which are not often covered by the legislation of a given country.[4]

Age and parity

Induced abortion is common when pregnancy is common. Numerically, women in their twenties have the most abortions. However, the social and economic pressures to restrict family size are strongest at the extremes of fertile life. A significant number of pregnancies in the young are conceived outside marriage. The phenomenon is most marked in industrialised nations, but is also emerging in the urban centres of some developing nations. For older women all over the world, economic, medical and, to some extent, emotional pressures to limit family size increase with age and parity. Therefore, although the proportion of abortions undergone by teenagers and women over 35 is always a minority of the overall total, the ratio of abortions to live births rises in these age groups.[5]

Marital status

Statistically the greater number of women who have abortions are married. Their prime motives for seeking abortions are the number of living children (and in some cultures the number of living sons) they already have and their socio-economic situation. In recent years there has been an increase in abortions among the young, married and unmarried, and a corresponding change in their motivation.[6]

On the one hand, in the West, the trend towards younger marriages has continued to accelerate, reversing the pattern of earlier centuries. Thus young couples are not always willing or able to assume the responsibilities of child-rearing immediately. On the other hand, the changing attitude towards sexual mores, greater freedom and education for women and freer social contacts between the sexes, cause men and women to have sexual experiences at an earlier age, whether married or not. Not all these young people, married or not, use contraceptives, and of those who do, not all use them effectively. For many, and increasingly the unmarried, abortion solves the problems of unwanted pregnancies and is looked upon as an alternative form of contraception. In most countries a certain social stigma is still attached to unwed motherhood, if not to the 'illegitimate' child. The unmarried, therefore, tend to resort to legal or illegal abortions regardless of the system. A change from a restricted to a moderate system probably would not distort this pattern unless there was a corresponding change in social attitudes toward the unmarried mother.[7]

Socio-economic factors

The education of women influences the abortion rate in a variety of ways, according to the culture of a country and the state of its development. Generally—but not universally—the higher the educational level of a woman, the greater is the tendency to seek an abortion to eliminate unwanted pregnancies either in the absence of contraception or to correct contraceptive failure.[8] Education encourages a more rational and purposeful attitude towards fertility. Thus, educated women are more apt to plan their families and to take concrete steps to limit the number of their children. On all levels, greater education of women is another aspect of the movement for female equality, and all over the world there is a strong correlation between advances in women's freedom and education and a belief in the woman's right to control the size of her family, whether with contraceptives or abortion.

Research in India found a strong correlation between education level and abortion rates: illiterate women report 3% of conceptions ending in abortions, those who receive middle grade education 9%, and high-school leavers 11%.[9] Possibly some levelling off in abortion rates is apparent amongst couples with university education for in this group 12% of conceptions end in abortions. Where demographic indicators are more established, as in Rio de Janeiro, the relationship can be the reverse—the higher socio-economic groups report an abortion rate one-tenth of that of the lowest groups.[10] This is probably due to improved sex education and availability of contraceptives. However, the figures suggest that in the case of contraceptive failure abortion is still resorted to.

Urban/rural differentials reflect socio-economic difficulties and in many developing countries the variation is gross—the variables separating the villager from the town dweller may be more significant than those separating comparable urban classes in developed and developing societies. The largest migration in human history is currently taking place as millions of people leave traditional village societies and move into the exploding cities of the Third World. The demographic experience of the historical shift towards urbanisation in Europe and North America differs from that of current trends in Asia and Africa. Nineteenth-century European urbanisation was accompanied by a rise in death rates, especially in infant mortality.[11] But now, modern and mass preventive medicine is so efficient that the killing diseases of the nineteenth-century cities are at least partially controlled, and adverse urban/rural differentials in infant mortality have been reduced or reversed.[12]

The chronic housing shortage in most of the cities of the world, the higher proportion of women working, often of necessity, the lack of centres to care for the children of working mothers and the impossibility of maintaining the extended family which could provide mother substitutes, have all made small families not an ideal but a necessity for urban couples. Large families can be a liability in the city, not only economically but in the time, energy and sheer physical space which parents must provide to raise them.

As an area becomes urbanised, there is an increasing use of abortion. Cities contain a large proportion of the poor who cannot afford to house, feed and educate large families; but they also have a strong representation of the upward-striving middle class with its stress on personal amenities, intensive education and also the strong belief that a child should be wanted and therefore planned. New city dwellers tend to adopt the patterns and mores of their new surroundings which favour small families. In Santiago in the 1960s women who had lived in the city for less than ten years had 13.3 induced abortions per 100 pregnancies, while those who had lived there for over ten years had 26.0.[13] Thus in the absence of contraception or in cases of contraceptive failure they turn to abortion. There seems less possibility of 'making do' with an extra, unwanted child in the cities than in the country.[14]

We can conclude that socio-economic factors are usually regarded as determinants of abortion rates. However, from a sociological point of view, Malcolm Potts, Peter Diggory and John Peel in their book, *Abortion,* assert that abortion must also be seen as a prime factor in socio-economic change. They argue that the differences in per capita income, education, literacy and female employment that characterise socio-economic advance are dependent on a reduction in achieved family size. They claim that no society has made such an adjustment without significant recourse to abortion—whether legal or illegal. Therefore, according to Potts, Diggory and Peel, induced abortion has been and is an intrinsic element in social and economic progress.[15] This assertion is based on a narrow interpretation of socio-economic development. An holistic approach to socio-economic change would view the recourse to abortion in a very different light.

Religion

In contrast to the influence exerted by socio-economic pressures, urbanisation and the need (or freedom) of women to work, the influence of religion on those who do not fully understand their faith appears slight. There may also be an understanding of their faith but a choice to disregard it when faced with a decision of whether to abort their child or not.

The power of traditional Catholicism has not prevented the implementation of liberal laws or the recourse to illegal abortions in Europe, the United States of America, Africa and certain Latin American countries. However certain studies have demonstrated some difference in the degree to which abortion is resorted to according to religious practice. The more devout and those better informed about their religious teachings are less likely to seek induced abortion than the indifferent or the uninstructed. However, when the general population was taken into account, the distinction of religious belief was similar in the abortion group to that in the total. The Lane Committee, reporting on the practice of abortion in the United Kingdom, found that despite the opposition of the Roman Catholic Church to abortion the percentage of Catholic women having abortions did not seem to be much lower than among fertile women in general. This led them to comment that, 'as with contraception, many women may be rejecting their Church's teaching in this field'.[16] These findings would appear to support the theory that couples set themselves well-defined goals of family size and, although they use different combinations of abortion and contraception to achieve these, in the last analysis no system of beliefs effectively deflects from abortion.

ABORTION IN THE JUDEO-CHRISTIAN TRADITION

An appreciation of the development of the Christian attitude towards abortion must take note not only of the biblical influences, but also of the philosophical understanding of the status of the embryo, medical science and the moral values of society in which it found itself. As medical science and philosophical understanding developed, so the attitude of the churches progressed.

In the Mediterranean world into which Christianity appeared, abortion was a familiar act. The reasons for abortion, according to Soranos of Ephesus (AD 98–138) were: to conceal the consequences of adultery; to maintain feminine beauty; and to avoid danger to the mother when her uterus was too small to accommodate the full embryo.[17] Abortion according to contemporary observers, was practised very generally in the Greco-Roman world. John Noonan puts forward the belief that the diminution of the Roman upper class during the Empire was probably due to their extensive practice of abortion and contraception.[18]

Christianity's attitude towards abortion would therefore be influenced by two traditions: the biblical tradition with its Middle Eastern roots and the philosophical understanding of the fetus that was current in the Greco-Roman world.

The biblical tradition has its roots in the civilisation of the Levant. The codes of Hammurabi, the Hittites and the Assyrians all prescribed compensation due for striking a woman so as to cause her to lose the child in her womb. The Hittites calculated this compensation on the gestational age of the fetus.[19] The Hebrew law on abortion comes from the Book of Exodus, and more specifically from that part of Exodus known as the book of the Covenant (20:22–23:19). It reads as follows:

> When, in the course of a brawl, a man knocks against a pregnant woman so that she has a miscarriage but suffers no further injury, then the offender must pay whatever fine the woman's husband demands after assessment. But where injury ensues, you are to give life for life, eye for eye, tooth for tooth, hand for hand, foot for foot, burn for burn, bruise for bruise, wound for wound.[20]

This is an example of what is called casuistic law, a model used frequently in the book of the Covenant.

More important for the development of subsequent Christian tradition than the Hebrew text is the Septuagint version of the same text. The Greek translation of the Bible produced in Alexandria in the third century before Christ carries a version of the text on abortion quite different from the Hebrew text cited above. It reads:

> If two men strive and smite a woman, and her child is imperfectly formed, he shall be forced to pay a penalty; as the woman's husband shall lay upon him, he shall pay with a valuation. But if he be perfectly formed, he shall give life for life.[21]

As can be seen the basic distinction made here regarding penalties differs considerably from that of the Hebrew text.

There the line was drawn between the death of the fetus (miscarriage) and the death of the mother (or other injury). In the Greek text the distinction is between the perfectly formed and imperfectly formed fetus. There is no reference to injury to the mother. The death penalty is imposed if the fetus is perfectly formed; otherwise an indemnity to be decided by the husband is prescribed. The implication here is that abortion of the formed fetus is considered homicide, whereas the abortion of the unformed fetus is penalised as something less than homicide. According to this version, the fetus is treated as a human being in the eyes of the law as soon as it is formed, not when it is born, as seemed to be the case in the Hebrew text.[22]

The older Latin versions of the Bible as well as St Jerome's Vulgate translation of the Hebrew text in the fourth century follows the Septuagint translation. It was these versions which formed the basis of canonical legislation in the Western Church. This was probably due to the prevailing philosophical understanding of the relation of body and soul, and with the physiological development in Hippocratic and Galenic medicine.[23]

The silence of the New Testament regarding abortion surpasses even that of the Old Testament. Yet it does teach basic values, such as the dignity of the person, protection of innocent life, the concept of parenthood and the commandment to love, on which the early Christian community grounded its arguments.[24]

Thus Paul in denouncing the foolish carnality of the Galatian community reminded them that there was a law which was fulfilled in one word, 'love your neighbour as yourself' (Gal. 5:14), and set out specific types of behaviour which violated it (Gal. 5:19–21). These included works of the flesh, which embraced not only 'lecheries' and 'wraths' but also *pharmakeia* (Gal. 5:20). *Pharmakeia* is a medicine or medicines with occultic properties used for a variety of purposes, including, in particular, contraception and abortion. Paul's usage of the word *pharmakeia* cannot be restricted to abortion only, but the term is comprehensive enough to include the use of abortifacient drugs.[25]

The Didache, an early Christian writing around AD 100, lists a group of precepts for the instruction of the Christian community. This includes commands not to practise 'medicine' (*pharmakeia*), to slay children by abortions (*phthora*), or to kill what is generated.[26] Thus, within the commandments concerning sexual sins, abortion was ranked as a principal sin and included in those expressly named ten commandments. Abortion was seen as an offence against God because it attacked what he had made. The *Epistle of Pseudo-Barnabas*[27] follows with a similar condemnation of abortion and infanticide.[28]

Early medieval observations, as found in the Hippocratic corpus, estimated that it took between thirty-five and fifty days for a fetus to become fully formed. These observations were to have a profound influence on the philosophical speculation on the status of the fetus. Aristotle argued that the earliest embryo had a vegetative existence animated[29] by a 'nutritive' soul; that the later embryo, resembling a little animal, had a 'sensitive' soul; and the formed fetus, recognisably human, a 'rational' or 'intellectual' soul. He links quickening and differentiation into distinct parts at 40 days for the male and 90 days for the female. This is the reason why traditionally he has been interpreted as placing the beginning of the individual male and female child at those times respectively. This is the origin of the period of 40 days after which the abortion of a fetus would be regarded morally as the equivalent of homicide. However, we know that Aristotle was mistaken in his account of the formation of the male after 40 days and the female after 90 days. By day 53 the external genitalia are still insufficiently developed for gender to be determined. It has been suggested that Aristotle probably mistook the remainder of the tail fold at day 40 for the penis. All normal embryos would have appeared in this way to be male, while those that were developing abnormally and did not show any part of the tail fold would have been considered female. In fact, it should be noted that a large proportion of embryos that are abnormal appear to be undifferentiated and are usually spontaneously aborted. By day 90 the genitalia are quite apparent. This is one plausible explanation for Aristotle's view

that boys are formed after 40 days and girls after 90 days.[30]
These were the limits within which, in the later moral tradition,
a fetus was held to be *formatus et animatus* (formed and
animated) and so indisputably human.

The Christian tradition tended to follow this distinction
between formed and unformed fetuses. However, two of the
early fathers appear to take a different approach. Tertullian, the
North African lawyer, in his *Apologia*, (which is a defence
against accusations that Christians sacrifice children), states that
Christians always held homicide to be wrong. He argues that
according to the law of Christ homicide is forbidden, therefore it
is not lawful to destroy what is conceived in the womb. He
denies the distinction between formed and unformed by saying
that it makes 'no difference whether you snatch away the soul
after birth or destroy it while coming to birth. Even the man who
is yet to be is a man, just as every fruit is already present in
seed.'[31]

This would appear to be an outright condemnation of any form
of abortion. Yet in his work *De Anima* in which abortion, or
rather dismemberment of the fetus, to save the life of the mother
is discussed, he argues that it is sometimes 'a cruel necessity' to
kill the fetus. The reason he gives is that without the death of the
fetus the mother herself will die.[32] This text appears to justify
embryotomy[33] to save the mother's life. Yet amongst scholars
there is some dispute on this interpretation. But what is evident
is that if he did approve of craniotomy[34] it was only as an
exception to his general condemnation of abortion for social
reasons.

Basil the Great (330–79) in a series of letters to Amphilochius,
Bishop of Iconium, follows Tertullian by writing that 'a woman
who deliberately destroys a fetus is answerable for murder. And
any fine distinction as to its being completely formed or
unformed is not admissible among us.'[35] The rigidity of Basil
and Tertullian appears to be at variance with the tradition in the
Western Church. St Gregory of Nysea (330–95) uses Basil's
distinction between formed and unformed embryos as the basis
for his theological reflection. He writes that it is not possible to

call an unformed embryo a human being, but only a potential one, because while it is in this unformed state it is something other than a human being. Therefore, according to Gregory, only a formed fetus can receive a soul.[36]

Similarly St Augustine of Hippo (354–430) follows this distinction in his theological arguments. 'If what is brought forth is unformed (*informe*) but at this stage some sort of living, shapeless thing (*informiter*), then the law of homicide would not apply, for it could not be said that there was a living soul in that body, for it lacks all sense, if it be such as is not yet formed (*nondum formata*) and therefore not yet endowed with its senses.'[37] This distinction between what was or was not homicide persisted throughout the centuries. It was to have a major influence in determining the canonical penalties for causing a miscarriage.[38]

An important development in the following centuries centred around cases of abortion where the mother's life was threatened. One observes in some authors a very narrow interpretation based solely on biological evidence, while in other authors the threat is perceived to include social conditions as well.

St Thomas follows the distinction between formed and unformed fetuses and the theological interpretation that only formed fetuses could be ensouled. He clearly states that it is actual homicide to kill an ensouled embryo.[39] Yet he was equally clear that ensoulment did not take place at conception.[40] Nevertheless, Thomas argued that it was sinful to destroy an unformed fetus, but the gravity of the act was less than killing a formed and ensouled fetus.[41] In his writings, St Thomas considered only one practical case of abortion, when it was for the child's own good. In this case the conflict is between the mother's life and that of the fetus. Pious zealots of Thomas's day proposed a caesarian section of the living woman, extraction of the near-term infant, and its baptism. Thus the child's life on earth and eternal salvation would be assured. The mother, of course, would die, but being baptised, her salvation would be secure. The advantage of this solution is that there would now be two souls in heaven and not one in heaven (mother's) and one in limbo (the unbaptised infant's). Thomas rejected the proposed new solution, on the explicit grounds that a caesarian section of a living woman would kill the mother.[42]

But what of abortion to save the mother? Thomas poses the question: 'Is it lawful for someone to kill *someone* in defending himself?' It should be noted that when Thomas wanted to characterise the one being killed he uses terms like 'sinner' and 'innocent'. Yet in this case he merely uses the word 'someone'. He answers the question by saying that, 'If someone kills someone in defence of his own life, he will not be guilty of homicide.' The act was lawful because 'what was intended was the preservation of one's own life'. The intention was not sinful, for it is 'natural to everyone to preserve himself as far as he can'. If it can be concluded that not all killing is forbidden and that an indifferent act may be justified by a good intention, could an argument be made for justifying abortion to save the life of the mother? This would depend on how absolutely Thomas meant his declaration, 'in no way is it lawful to kill the innocent', which is made in other contexts. If this principle were applied absolutely it would preclude capital punishment for a person who had repented his or her crime; yet Thomas justifies capital punishment. The principle would also have precluded many acts of warfare such as killing enemy soldiers in good faith, or killing infants in attacking fortresses, acts which Thomas condones. Authors like John Noonan conclude that from Thomas's writings it cannot be said definitively that he justified therapeutic abortions to save the mother's life.[43] Other authors, however, interpret Thomas as justifying therapeutic abortions if the mother's life were in danger.

Between 1450 and 1750 a number of attempts were made, by moralists, to strike a balance between the life of the early conceptus and the life of the woman. The Spanish Jesuit Tomas Sanchez (1550–1610) was the first moralist to attempt a theological defence of therapeutic abortion. While arguing that there was an absolute prohibition on contraception, he held there were exceptions to the prohibition of abortions. In instances in which the mother would otherwise die, and the fetus was not ensouled, its killing was 'more probably' lawful.[44] The justification was that the intention of the woman was to save her own life, an act which had the double effect of taking the life of the fetus and preserving the life of the woman. But it was the intention of the woman, rather than the *de facto* end result of the act—the killing of the fetus—which was, in Sanchez's view, decisive. He also considered two cases in which the threat to the woman's life came not directly from the fetus, but the social consequences of pregnancy which could be considered life threatening. If a woman had conceived outside marriage and there was a threat to her life if her family discovered this, could she kill the fetus? Sanchez thought it probable that she could. In another case, if a woman already betrothed became pregnant by someone other than her intended husband and found that the engagement could not be terminated without a scandal could she kill the fetus to avert the danger of scandal and also to ensure that she did not bear a child to a man who was not its father? Sanchez believed she could. What becomes apparent in Sanchez's arguments is that other values, like paternity and social values, were allowed to be weighed against the embryo's life. Sanchez is credited by some authors as having proposed the first non-medical grounds for therapeutic abortion.[45]

St Alfonso de Liguori addressed the question under the general heading, 'Is it sometimes licit to kill the innocent?' and under the specific heading 'Is it sometimes lawful to procure an abortion?' He held that Sanchez's opinion permitting the intentional killing of the unformed fetus to save the mother was a probable opinion, but that the 'more common opinion' held that as it was never licit to expel the seed, even in rape, 'so much less is it lawful to expel the fetus which is closer to human life.' The more common opinion was 'safer' and therefore to be followed. Like Sanchez, Liguori introduced the distinction of means 'tending directly' to kill the fetus, such as blows and wounding, and held these illicit, while 'indirect' treatment to save the mother like the cutting of the mother's veins, purging of her body, and baths were permissible. Moreover, the threat to the mother's life had to be immediate. Therefore abortion, if there was a danger of being killed by irate relatives, was not justifiable. With these reservations, therapeutic abortion to save the mother from immediate danger was permitted; the intention to save her own life must predominate; only some means were permitted. The balance struck by the casuists and set out by St Alfonso treated the embryo's life as less than absolute, but only the value of the mother's own life was given greater weight.[46]

With St Alfonso, what might be called the classic period of moral theology came to an end. After him one would no longer see the publication of multidimensional treatises of folio dimensions. Many more abbreviated works of manual size began to appear, and in fact many of them were no more than compendia of Alfonso's *Theologia moralis*. Generally speaking, the moral theologians of the late eighteenth and nineteenth centuries were heavily dependent upon his work and some did little more than repeat his opinion. But a number of significant developments did take place during this time which were to affect the legislation and theology on abortion. The move, pioneered by medical science, away from delayed animation and in the direction of immediate animation without distinction of sex, meant that new issues had to be dealt with. With the general acceptance, at least on the level of ecclesiastical practice and theological opinion, of immediate animation, the discussion of abortion of an inanimate fetus to save the mother lost all practical meaning. But the problem of dangerous pregnancy did not go away. If it was to be discussed now, however, it had to be in terms of the animated fetus. Therefore the problem of abortion of the animated fetus to save the mother's life, together with the related problem of craniotomy and embryotomy, would occupy moral theologians during the second half of the nineteenth century and would lead to the fine distinctions of the 'double effect theory' of the twentieth century.

ROMAN CATHOLIC ECCLESIAL LEGISLATION AND TWENTIETH-CENTURY PAPAL TEACHING

The publication in 1140 of Gratian's *Decretum* was the first fully systematic attempt to compile ecclesiastical legislation on abortion. He maintained the distinction which had occurred between the fifth and twelfth century, the distinction between formed and unformed fetus.[47] In answer to the question of whether those who procured abortions were guilty of homicide, Gratian reasons that it is not murder to abort a fetus before the soul is in the body. Gregory IX in 1235 with his *Decretals* sustained this position, but adds an ambiguous note. The *Decretals* included both the *Sicut Ex* canon, which contained Gratian's distinction, and another canon *Si Aliquis*, dating from the tenth century, which had specified that the penalty for homicide was to be applied to contraception and abortion, regardless of fetal development. The implicit contradiction between the two canons was soon taken to mean that while all abortions were murder, the canonical penalties (especially for clerics involved in abortions) should vary according to the stage of fetal life.[48]

Up until the sixteenth century and the reforming papacy of Pope Sixtus V the church followed a tradition which measured culpability with the development of the fetus. The Sacred Penitentiary did not treat as homicide the killing of an embryo under forty days. Even where the embryo over forty days was sinfully destroyed, the Penitentiary made less difficulty about dispensations than when an adult human was killed. This was not because they believed the older embryo to be subhuman, but that an embryo was rarely killed in hatred. The cases regularly involved women who had conceived in fornication and aborted the fetus to protect their reputations; and men who counselled them to do so in order to save their own reputations. Thus the protection of reputation was seen as extenuating circumstances.[49]

According to Sixtus V the practice of abortion had become such a problem to the church during the Renaissance that it was necessary for the church authority to legislate special penalties against it. Therefore on 29 October 1588 in his bull *Effraenatum* he abolished the traditional distinction between formed/animated and unformed/inanimate fetuses, and called all acts of abortion murder.[50] He also attached an excommunication not only to the pregnant woman, but also to anyone who would give advice, assistance, a potion, or any other kind of medication for the commissioning of this crime. The excommunication was extended to include the giving or taking of potions to induce sterility or to prevent conception. Absolution from the penalty was also reserved to the supreme pontiff, except when the one who had procured it was in danger of death.

Effraenatum was not an unqualified success. Not only was the reservation of absolution to the Holy See seen to be unworkable, but the departure from ecclesiastical precedents of distinguishing between animated and unanimated fetus clashed with the practice of the Sacred Penitentiary and the theory of canonists and theologians.

As a result, the next Pope, Gregory XIV, was quick to modify it. In the bull *Sedes Apostolica*, 31 May 1591, he stated:

The penalties for procuring the abortion of an inanimate fetus or for administering or taking potions to cause women to be sterile, we revoke just as if that constitution, so far as it concerns these things had never been issued.[51]

This meant that the excommunication for an abortion of the unanimated fetus and for sterilisation was withdrawn; it was limited to the abortion of the animated fetus. Also, absolution from the excommunication was no longer reserved to the supreme pontiff but could be given by the local bishop or anyone delegated by him. The constitution remained in effect for almost three centuries, being revised only in 1869 by Pius IX.

By the nineteenth century abortion, because of improved medical practice and a mood of population control defended in popular and scholarly literature, had increased. Against this current in favour of abortion the Roman Catholic Church reacted. Already by the nineteenth century the Aristotelian interpretation of gestation, which supposed a transformation from vegetable soul to rational soul occurring in the embryo, had become obsolete. This was mainly due to discoveries in medical science, commencing with Karl Ernst von Baer's discovery of the ovum in the human female. By the middle of the nineteenth century the joint action of spermatozoon and ovum in generation had been determined and accepted.

Therefore the proclamation of the dogma of the Immaculate Conception in 1854 by Pope Pius IX which stated that Mary was free from sin 'in the first instant of her conception'[52] was a major blow to both the traditional theological and biological development of the Aristotelian 'forty-day-eighty-day' formula.[53]

In 1869, in the constitution *Apostolicae Sedis*, Pius IX dropped all references to the distinction between unanimated and animated. The legislation seemed to include excommunication for the abortion of any fetus.[54] In the light of this document the Holy Office in a number of its judgments turned back even the most appealing exceptions to do with saving the mother's life in favour of the inviolability and independent integrity of the embryo. This legislation continued through subsequent pontificates and was incorporated in the *Code of Canon Law* published in 1917.[55] This still prevails in the church. The 1983 revised code maintains this excommunication:[56] 'A person who procures a completed abortion incurs excommunication *latae sententiae*',[57] 'by the very commission of the offence',[58] and subject to the conditions provided by Canon Law.[59] According to the *Universal Catechism* the church does not thereby intend to restrict the sense of mercy. Rather, she makes clear the gravity of the crime committed, the irreparable harm done to the innocent who is put to death, as well as to the parents and the whole of society.[60]

However, it should be noted that this is legislation, not teaching. Distinctions the church makes, or does not make, in regard to penalties do not constitute church teaching. So while it is true that the church today penalises abortion at any stage, it would be wrong to conclude from this that it teaches immediate animation or infusion of a rational soul in the fetus. This has never been the case.

This position was re-enforced by Pius XI in his encyclical *Casti connubii* issued in 1930. Although this encyclical was preoccupied with the problem of contraception, it touched briefly on abortion, even though little was said at that time about

abortion as a method of birth control. The encyclical spoke of
'that most grave crime of which the offspring hidden in the
maternal breast is attacked'. Speaking first of those who
justified it by medical and therapeutic indications, the Pope
asked, 'What cause can ever avail to excuse in any way the
direct killing of the innocent? For it is a question of that.
Whether it is inflicted on mother or on offspring, it is against
the commandment of God and the voice of nature, "You shall
not kill. The life of each is sacred".' The argument that the
mother could treat the fetus as an unjust aggressor did not apply,
'for who will call an innocent little one an unjust aggressor?'
The encyclical overruled writers like Sanchez by simply stating
that 'there is a law of extreme necessity which can lead to direct
killing of the innocent'.[61] Second the encyclical described as
wicked and 'lustful cruelty' those who practised abortion in
marriage to prevent offspring.[62] Finally the encyclical
condemned those advocating abortion on social and eugenic
grounds. It stated that the 'killing of the innocent' for such
reasons was 'contrary to the divine commandment promulgated
also by the words of the Apostle, 'evils are not to be done in
order that good comes from them.'[63] The independent destiny of
the fetus is not to be destroyed for its own good or the good of
others, was thus asserted.

Pope Pius XII, in a series of allocutions, frequently spoke on
the subject. In 1944 he said to the Italian Medical-Biological
Union of St Luke that as long as a person does not commit a
crime, his or her life is untouchable. Therefore 'every action
which tends directly towards its destruction is illicit', no matter
whether this life is embryonic or already approaching full
term.[64] Again in an address to the Italian Catholic Society of
Midwives on 29 October 1951 he taught that 'the being in the
maternal breast has the right to life immediately from God'.
There is no human authority, no science, no medical, eugenic,
social, economic or moral 'indicators' which can establish or
grant a valid juridical ground for a direct deliberate disposition
of an innocent human life, that is a disposition which looks to
its destruction either as an end or as a means to another end

perhaps in itself licit. The baby, still not born, is a person in the same degree and for the same reason as the mother is.[65]

Pius XII's successor, John XXIII, carried forward these themes. In *Mater et Magistra* (1961), he wrote that 'human life is sacred: from the very inception, the creative action of God is directly operative. By violating his laws, the Divine Master is offended, the individuals themselves and humanity degraded, and likewise the community itself of which they are members is enfeebled.'[66]

The Second Vatican Council was quite explicit in what it had to say about the value of life from the beginning:

Life must be safeguarded with the utmost care from the moment of conception; abortion and infanticide are abominable crimes.[67]

The reason given for the careful wording of this statement was to avoid 'the difficult question of the moment at which the soul is infused'.[68] In this declaration the Council made several doctrinal advances. For the first time contraception was treated differently from abortion. In condemning abortion no final judgment was made on all forms of contraception. Beyond these distinctions, an amendment, specifically made and adopted, added the words, 'from its conception'. In this way the Council sharply marked off the status of the conceptus from the status of spermatozoa and ova. Finally, the declaration was the first statement ever made by a General Council of the church on abortion; its judgments represented a commitment by the Catholic bishops of the world to care for the conceptus.

After the Vatican Council, Pope Paul VI, in his encyclical on birth control, *Humanae Vitae* (1968), said that once again the church must declare that 'the direct interruption of the generative process already begun, and, above all, directly willed and procured abortion, even if for therapeutic reasons, are to be absolutely excluded as licit means of regulating birth'.[69]

This teaching is taken up and explained in much greater detail by the Congregation for the Doctrine of the Faith in its

Declaration on Procured Abortion. Although appealing to Scripture and tradition the document also demonstrates that its arguments make sense in the light of human reason. It argues that respect for human life is called for from the time that the process of generation begins. 'From the time that the ovum is fertilised, a life is begun which is neither that of the father nor of the mother; it is rather the life of a new human being with its own growth.'[70] It goes on to argue that the moment of animation has no bearing on the discussion. Rather it points out that modern genetic science demonstrates that from the first instant there is established the programme of what this living being will be: a person. The *Declaration* then goes on to state that it is not up to biological science to make definitive judgments on questions that are in fact philosophical and moral, such as the moment when a human person is constituted or on the legitimacy of abortion. Finally, it argues that even if there is a doubt concerning whether the conceptus is already a human person, it is 'objectively a grave sin to dare to risk murder'.[71] Although not formally teaching that there is a full human life present from the moment of fertilisation, the document, owing to the 'risk of murder', rules out all abortions regardless of the stage of fetal development. This is stated more forcefully in the Apostolic See's *Chapter of the Rights of the Family*: 'Human life must be respected and protected absolutely from the moment of conception.'[72]

Owing to speculation regarding the status of the embryo raised by the increasing practice of in vitro fertilisation and experimentation, the Congregation for the Doctrine of the Faith felt it necessary to re-state the Catholic teaching in its *Instruction on Respect for Human Life in Its Origin and on the Dignity of Procreation.* Drawing substantially on the 1974 document, *Declaration on Procured Abortion*, its arguments can be summarised in four stages. First, the life of the fertilised ovum is neither that of the father nor that of the mother, it is a *new* life. Second, this new life is a *human* life, for it could not be made human if it were not human already. Third, this new human life is the life of an *individual*, for *identity or individuality* is established from the first instant. Finally, this *new human individual*, which comes into existence at the moment of conception, must surely be a person.[73] Following a strategy of safety, the Roman Catholic Church, once again, reiterates its teaching that any risk of directly killing a full human being must be avoided. It, therefore, regards its absolute prohibition on direct abortion as definitive and unchangeable.

Pope John Paul II has surpassed all of his predecessors in his references to induced abortion as something absolutely to be condemned. In general audiences, in familiar talks, as at the midday Angelus, in addressing the Cardinals or various hierarchies, in homilies during his various missionary journeys and in his encyclicals, he has reaffirmed the fundamental theme of the inviolability of human life from the moment of conception.

Rather than examining all the Pope's statements on this issue it will be useful to highlight those texts in which he outlines his personal theme. In these encyclicals abortion is seen in the perspective of his vision of the redeemed universe struggling still in the throes of its new birth until all its evil is cleansed in its final redemptive liberation: this liberation will not be until, amongst other things, strife amongst people, monstrous injustice and lack of reverence for human life, including its nascent stages, are wiped out.

Redemptor hominis (4 March 1979) recalls the magnificent vision of St Paul of the renewal of all creation in Christ the Redeemer, which nonetheless expects impatiently 'the revelation of the sons of God', being as yet 'subject to vanity'.[74] For Pope John Paul this vanity is particularly conspicuous at the present time when people's domination of the material world has brought with it a host of evils: contamination of the atmosphere, the continuing and increasing arms race, the possibility of human extinction by ourselves through the employment of atomic, hydrogen, neutron bombs and other similar weapons, and 'decreasing reverence for the life of the unborn'.[75]

Dives in misericordia (30 November 1980) sees the preoccupation and anxiety of modern people as due to a certain lack of sensibility to fundamental moral values, to which we must be attuned by love rather than by justice alone. Such values are the heritage not only of Christian morality but of sound humanity and its moral culture. Amongst them is respect for human life from the moment of conception.[76]

In the encyclical *Veritatis splendor* (6 August 1993) the Pope gives the foundations of morality. In the chapter entitled the 'Moral Act' and the sub-section concerned with 'intrinsic evil' abortion is condemned as an act which is *per se* and in itself, independent of circumstances, always seriously wrong by reason of the object.[77]

These references to abortion, although brief in some documents, go to the heart of the papal teaching. Abortion is a blot, an ugly chasm on the mounting horizon of human redemption in Christ; it is a savage act of cruelty towards a helpless human, in flagrant contradiction to the mercy of the Creator. The Pope's vision is whole, clear and penetrating. He argues that if a person's right to life is violated at the moment in which he or she is first conceived in the mother's womb, an indirect blow is struck at the whole moral order, which serves to ensure the inviolable goods of the person. Among these goods life occupies the primal position. The church, therefore, defends the right to life, not only because God is the Creator, but also in respect of the essential good of the human person.[78] The Pope concludes by pointing out that the denial of the right to life of the newly conceived undermines the entire fabric of Christian and natural morality.

The *Catechism* reiterates this tradition by stating that:

Human life must be respected and protected absolutely from the moment of conception. From the first moment of his existence, a human being must be recognised as having the rights of a person—among which is the inviolable right of every innocent being to life.[79]

It goes on to argue that the 'inalienable right to life of every innocent individual is a constitutive element of a civil society

and its legislation'.[80] It stresses the point that if these rights are
not upheld then the very foundations of a state based on law are
undermined.[81]

In his encyclical, *Evangelium Vitae* (25 March 1995), Pope
John Paul II once again sets out to uphold and defend the
sanctity of human life and more specifically to censure those
who believe in abortion. The encyclical's novelty lies largely in
the vividness of its language and the finality attached to its
definitive edicts. These are dramatically presented within a
framework of an underlying conflict between two cultures: the
'culture of life' and the 'culture of death'. The style and tone of
the encyclical prepares the reader for an infallible
pronouncement which does not occur. However, this was
evidently not the original intention. According to the Italian
journalist Lucio Brunelli the explicit references to infallible
teaching were removed immediately prior to sending the
encyclical to the printers, the reason being that John Paul II did
not want to go down in history as the first pope to break the
tradition whereby popes only define matters of faith as dogmas,
not matters of morals.[82]

The Pope begins by asserting that the *Gospel of Life* is both a
great gift of God and an exacting task for humanity. It gives rise
to amazement and gratitude in the person graced with freedom,
and it asks to be welcomed, preserved and esteemed, with a deep
sense of responsibility. 'In giving life to man, God demands that
he love, respect and promote life. The gift thus becomes a
commandment, and the commandment is itself a gift.'[83]
Therefore, people are understood to be 'ministers of God's plan'
and are entrusted to ensure that life is treasured and not
squandered. Arising from this understanding he teaches that the
scriptural commandment 'You shall not kill' has absolute value
when it refers to the innocent person. The sacredness and
inviolability of human life has been taught consistently by the
church's Magisterium. However, due to the progressive
weakening of both individual and social conscience on the
absolute and grave illicitness of the direct taking of all innocent
human life John Paul declares that by 'the authority which Christ

conferred upon Peter and his Successors, and in communion with the Bishops of the Catholic Church, I confirm that the direct and voluntary killing of an innocent human being is always gravely immoral.'[84]

When referring explicitly to abortion the Pope argues that today, in many people's consciences, the perception of its gravity has become progressively obscured. The acceptance of abortion in the popular mind, in behaviour and even in law itself, is a telling sign of an extremely dangerous crisis of the moral sense, which is becoming more and more incapable of distinguishing good and evil, even when the fundamental right to life is at stake. He therefore declares that abortion must be recognised for what it actually is. Procured abortion is 'the deliberate and direct killing, by whatever means it is carried out, of a human being in the initial phase of his or her existence, extending from conception to birth'.[85] He recognises that the decision to have an abortion is often a tragic and painful one for the mother, made neither for purely selfish reasons nor out of convenience, but out of a desire to protect certain important values such as her own health or a decent standard of living for the other members of the family. Nevertheless, these reasons and others like them, however serious and tragic, 'can never justify the deliberate killing of an innocent human being'.[86] John Paul goes on to declare that 'direct abortion, that is, abortion willed as an end or as a means, always constitutes a grave moral disorder, since it is the deliberate killing of an innocent human being'.[87] This doctrine, he maintains, is based upon natural law and upon the written Word of God, which is transmitted by the church's tradition and taught by the ordinary and universal Magisterium. No circumstances, no purpose, no law whatsoever can ever make licit an act which is intrinsically illicit, since it is contrary to the Law of God which is written in every human heart, knowable by reason itself and proclaimed by the church.[88]

There is no doubt that the absolutist position of the present Pope and of papal teaching this century is expressed with rigorous philosophical consistency and power. But moral absolutism of this type can be a liability as well as a strength.

The distance between the absolutist preacher and the practical legislator can become unbridgeable and, as a result, the voice of idealism is rejected altogether. On abortion, that is a line the Pope is dangerously near to crossing. All over the world, most recently in Ireland, Roman Catholic legislators have been turning their backs on papal absolutism to pass laws to permit their citizens some access to abortion. They recognise what the *Evangelium Vitae* denies: that the civil law must sometimes compromise for the greater good, not least to make room for those who do not wish to subscribe to Roman Catholic teaching.[89]

ROMAN CATHOLIC THEOLOGICAL UNDERSTANDING

Four basic principles summarise the Roman Catholic theological position on abortion. They are: God alone is the Lord of life and death; human beings do not have the right to take the lives of other innocent human beings; human life begins at the moment of conception; and abortion, at whatever the stage of development of the conceptus, is the taking of innocent human life.

The primary principle that *God alone is the Lord of life and death* has its foundation in the Christian principle of the 'sanctity of human life'. According to the Protestant theologian Paul Ramsey the value of a human life is ultimately grounded in the value God places on it.[90] From this two points emerge. First, in the religious view, the sanctity of human life is not a function of the worth any human being may attribute to it; this therefore precludes discussion of any 'degrees of relative worth' a human being may have or acquire. Second, Ramsey wants to make clear that a person's life 'is entirely an ordination, a loan, and a stewardship. His essence is his existence before God and to God, and it is from Him.'[91] In this formulation, a person must respect his or her own life and the lives of others not only because it is grounded in God, but, equally important, because God has given a person life as a value to be held in trust and used according to God's will. Catholic theology is parallel to Protestant theology in emphasising God as the source and ultimate guarantor of the sanctity of human life. Thus Josef Fuchs asserts that 'man as such belongs directly and exclusively to God'.[92] Norman St John-Stevas, who has written extensively on this subject, argues that 'respect for the lives of others because of their eternal destiny is the essence of the Christian teaching. Its other aspect is the emphasis on the creatureliness of a person. A person is not absolutely master of his or her own life and body. He or she has no *dominium* over it, but holds it in trust for God's purposes.[93] St John-Stevas goes on to contend that the sanctity of life is a fundamental principle which has sustained Western society, the rejection or dilution of which would endanger the whole of human life, and that, in any case, there is no other principle available which would provide a 'criterion of the right to life, save that of personal taste'.[94]

Therefore, central to both Catholic and Protestant theology is the principle that God is the Lord of life and death.[95] This is another way of proclaiming that a person holds his or her life in trust, of asserting that a person's ultimate value stems from God and of saying that no person can take it upon themselves to place themselves in total mastery over the life of another. To confess that God is Lord of life and death is to affirm that a person is a creature, owing his or her existence, his or her value and his or her ultimate destiny to God.[96] This basic premise will be resorted to continually in Catholic moral theology in determining the morality of in vitro fertilisation, genetics and euthanasia.

The second principle is that *human beings do not have the right to take the lives of other innocent human beings*. This proposition is consistent with Christian ethics and the Catholic natural-law morality. The word 'innocent', however, is crucial. Traditional Catholic morality has defended the just war theory and capital punishment. Wars have been justified even though they result, often enough, in the foreseen taking of innocent life, particularly the life of non-combatants. The justification of this taking of innocent life, however, is governed by the principle of the double effect. Thus innocent life cannot be taken unless, for the strict demands of self-defence, these lives are taken only 'indirectly', that is, by an action 'designed and intended solely to achieve some other purpose(s) even though death is foreseen as a concomitant effect. Death therefore is not positively willed, but is reluctantly permitted as an unavoidable by-product.'[97] Thus, while the proposition concerning the absence of the right of one human being to take the life of another is basic to Catholic morality, it admits of an important exception in two cases: when the life to be taken is not innocent human life and when it is 'innocent' life but the taking of that life is 'indirect'.

The third principle, *human life begins at the moment of conception*, is a re-affirmation of Pius IX's judgment that the traditional distinction between a formed and unformed fetus is no longer applicable in the case of abortion. The question of when human life begins and the problem of whether an early embryo should be considered a human with potential or a potential human will be dealt with in more detail in the chapter on in vitro fertilisation. Nevertheless, it is sufficient to say that the Catholic Church has never officially taught when the individual human being, endowed with a rational soul, begins in the mother's womb.[98] This point is aptly demonstrated in the 1974 *Declaration on Procured Abortion* which argues that 'respect for human life is called for from the time that the process of generation begins. From the time that the ovum is fertilised, a life is begun which is neither that of the father nor of the mother; it is rather the life of a new human being (*novi viventis humani*) with his own growth. It would never be made human if it were not human already.'[99] The church stopped short of categorically asserting that the fertilised egg itself is already a human being or a person. An important footnote to paragraph 13 makes this clearer.[100] The *Declaration* therefore does not intend to resolve the point of the moment of spiritual or rational ensoulment. Rather the church recognises that this is still an ongoing biological, philosophical and theological debate.[101] Richard McCormick concludes that while this discussion continues, the benefit of the doubt should be given to the embryo.[102] This is precisely what the church in her condemnation of all abortions has done.

The fourth principle follows easily once the question of

whether the conceptus from the moment of conception is 'human life' has been answered in the affirmative. This principle states that *abortion, at whatever the stage of development of the conceptus, is the taking of innocent human life.*

With these premises as a basis it is not difficult to understand why many Catholics view with alarm the prospect of a moral acceptance of abortion. Therefore, if the act of abortion is the killing of an innocent human being it demands that it must be vigorously opposed.

This has led many Catholic theologians to believe that since theology is confronted with a clear and unchangeable doctrine of the ordinary magisterium, there remains only the necessity of explaining clearly the reasons behind the doctrine and discussing whether some complicated cases might be considered as 'indirect abortions'. These are normally dealt with under the principle of double effect. For it to be applicable at least four conditions must be met: (i) the act must itself be either good or indifferent, or at least not forbidden with a view to preventing just that effect; (ii) the evil effect cannot be a means to the good, but must be equally immediate or at least must result from the good effect; (iii) the foreseen evil effect must not be intended or approved, merely permitted—for even a good act is vitiated if accompanied by an evil intent; (iv) there must be a proportionately serious reason for exercising the cause of allowing the evil effect.[103] Therefore the classic two exceptions: abortion in the instance of an ectopic pregnancy and the instance of a cancerous uterus fulfil these criteria.

Pius XII approved the rationale for these exceptions when in 1951 he argued that if the saving of the life of the future mother, independently of her pregnant condition, required a surgical act or other therapeutic treatment which would have as an accessory consequence, in no way desired or intended, but inevitable, the death of the fetus, such an act could no longer be called a direct attempt on an innocent life. Under these conditions the operation would be lawful, provided that a 'good of high worth' was concerned, such as life, and that it was not possible to postpone the operation until after the birth of the child, nor to have access to other efficacious remedies.[104] Similarly the problem of an ectopic pregnancy also illustrated a legitimate use of the principle. In this instance it is proposed that the removal of a non-viable fetus from the fallopian tube, before the external rupture of the tube, could be done in such a way that the consequent death of the fetus would be produced only indirectly. Such an operation could be licitly performed if all the circumstances were such that the necessity for the operation were, in moral estimation, proportionate to the evil effect permitted.[105] In this instance, the intention of the operation itself is good (as a standard operation to save life); although the fetus is killed, that effect, though foreseen, is not the intention of the operation (thus the death of the fetus is indirectly caused); the evil effect (the death of the fetus) is not the means to the good end (the saving of the life of the woman), but only the indirect result of the means (the tubal removal) necessary to save the life of the woman. Thus the conditions for an application of the principle are met. By contrast a fetal craniotomy to save the life of the woman would not be licit because, in that case, the life of the fetus is taken directly by the act of crushing its skull. The intention is good (saving the life of the woman), but the means employed are evil (directly taking the life of an innocent fetus); therefore fetal craniotomy is forbidden.[106]

In reaction to the rigidity of the application of the double effect theory, Daniel Callahan argues that it places an undue emphasis on the physical life alone as the only value at stake, leaving no room for even investigating any other considerations which might come into play. He contends that the real interest in the extreme case of letting both woman and fetus die turns out, in effect, not to be the good of the mother, but the good conscience of those who might but do not act to save her. Therefore, the basic moral principle of 'Do good and avoid evil' is now rendered into avoiding evil alone.[107]

A more systematic critique of the Catholic approach, which is characterised by establishing general principles from which specific applications are made, is offered by Protestant theologian James Gustafson. He points out that the arguments are *externally juridical*, that is they are written from the perspective of people who claim the right to judge the past actions of others as morally right or wrong, or to tell others what future actions are morally right or wrong. Second, a *juridical model* is applied. The action is either right or wrong depending on whether it conforms to or is contrary to a rule or a law. Third, traditional Catholic arguments are largely confined to the relevant *physical* data. The concern is primarily with physical life, its sanctity and its preservation. It is obvious that other aspects of human life depend upon the biological basis of the human body, and the primacy of this concern is valid up to a point. But on the whole, the arguments have not been extended to include a concern for the emotional and spiritual well-being of the mother or infant. The concern is mainly with the physical consequences of abortion, and little thought is given to the emotional or spiritual consequences of bringing a pregnancy to term. Gustafson's fourth point highlights the fact that Roman Catholic arguments limit themselves almost *exclusively to the physician and patient* at the time of pregnancy, without giving due regard to the multiple relationships and responsibilities each has to and for others over a long period of time. His fifth point is that Catholic arguments are too *rationalistic*. This tends to reduce the spiritual and personal individuality of each person to abstract cases. The sense of human compassion for suffering and profound tragedy which is built into any situation in which the taking of life is morally plausible, are gone. His final point criticises the belief that arguments based on the *natural law* ought to be persuasive and binding on all of humanity. This does not give due recognition to other serious thinkers who have rejected the natural law theory and resorted to other ethical criteria as the basis of their moral judgments.[108]

THEOLOGICAL DEVELOPMENT BY SOME ROMAN CATHOLIC THEOLOGIANS

Various approaches to the morality of abortion tend to dominate the present discussion. I have decided to deal with only three of these approaches as they represent some of the main schools of thought. Unfortunately many interesting and worthy contributions made by leading theologians will have to be neglected. The following approaches will, one hopes, introduce the reader to the rich debate which still continues within Roman Catholic theological circles. The first approach could be termed the individualistic method which has an almost exclusive dependence on biological and physical criteria. Second, there is the relational approach which is unwilling to accept just physical criteria and argues for more personalistic criteria in assessing the beginning of life. Finally, there is an effort to broaden the traditional understanding of the 'double effect theory' and to respond to the pastoral situation.

The individualistic or generic method attempts to determine from physical or biological evidence the presence of a human individual. As has been seen, traditional Catholic theology teaches that this begins at conception. However, Joseph Donceel S.J., who has written often on the subject, espouses a theory of delayed animation that, in his judgment, is the teaching proposed by St Thomas Aquinas. This theory is not based on Thomas's admittedly inaccurate biological knowledge, but on his philosophical theory of hylomorphism.[109] According to this theory, the soul is the substantial form of the body, but a substantial form can only be present in matter capable of receiving it. The fertilised ovum or early embryo, because they are not fully formed, cannot have a human soul. A human being's spiritual faculties have no organs of their own, but the activity of cogitative power presupposes that the being be fully developed, that the cortex be formed. While admitting that he is uncertain as to when a human soul is infused into matter, Donceel nevertheless proposes rather strict criteria to judge animation. He suggests that the senses, the nervous system, the brain and particularly the cortex be formed before admitting the presence of a human soul. Since these organs are not fully formed in early pregnancy, he feels certain that there is no human person until several weeks have elapsed.[110] This perception of animation obviously affects Donceel's understanding of abortion. Leading him to conclude that although a 'prehuman embryo' cannot demand the absolute respect which we owe to the human person, it deserves a very great consideration, because it is a living being, individual with a human finality, on its way to hominisation. Therefore, he holds that 'only very serious reasons should allow us to terminate its existence'.[111] What these reasons are Donceel does not say. However, he does seem to imply that they would be broader than the traditional ones applied in the double effect theory.

John Mahoney S.J., although not specifically referring to abortion, supports this understanding of delayed animation. Due to the facts of actual or possible twinning and combination of fertilised eggs, he argues, that rather than ensoulment occurring at the stage of conception, it can take place only when there is an unambiguously individual subject capable of receiving the soul by virtue of the fact that it has passed beyond the stage of simple reduplication and has begun to ramify and diversify through the development of its bodily organs.[112]

In a similar way Fr Norman Ford, in his book *When Did I Begin?*, argues that it is only possible to speak of a human individual when the primitive streak occurs. For about 14 days after fertilisation, until the appearance of the primitive streak, the multiplying cells are naturally synthesising a human individual.[113] He also suggests that natural indicators should also be utilised to determine when individual human life has commenced. Nature's own sign to a woman that she may be pregnant is her first missed menses after sexual intercourse: this would usually occur about two weeks after fertilisation. This is the time when the primitive streak would have appeared after implantation had taken place. It might, therefore, be possible to acknowledge the suggestion by certain biologists that implantation should be taken as conception.[114] Although Ford does not deal explicitly with abortion his research and conclusions have important implications for how we view the moral acceptability of abortifacient contraceptives. In traditional Roman Catholic morality they were perceived as immoral because they killed the conceptus which was considered to be innocent human life. If, as Donceel and Ford suggest, this is not the case then perhaps the immorality of these abortifacient devices needs to be re-assessed.

An unwillingness to accept simply biological criteria for determining when human life begins, and its implications for abortion, is a characteristic of the relational school of theology. This school bases its arguments on the centrality of acceptance and recognition by the parents. Jacques-Marie Pohier turns to the anthropological evidence of certain societies and tribes where the decision to accept the child into their society is made after birth. Although he disagrees with this approach he nevertheless argues that it does demonstrate how essential the relational aspect of acceptance is for truly human life.[115] Parents by their acceptance of the fetus, especially through naming it, make the fetus a subject who has a place in this world. It is not a child until the decision of the parents anticipates the human form and begin to speak of it as a human subject.[116] Following from this thesis Bruno Ribes asserts that where the relationship between the infant and the parents does not exist now or will not exist at birth, one has the duty to ask about the legitimacy of allowing such a child to be born.[117]

Certain authors within the relational school insist that the fact that many people in contemporary society do not have moral difficulties in terminating a pregnancy, for a variety of broad reasons, must be taken seriously. Bernard Quelquejeu calls for an entirely new theological methodology in the light of such experience. He argues that one can no longer begin with established moral principles and apply them to these different situations, but rather one must begin with the moral experience as manifest in these different decisions. The experience of women who decide to have an abortion definitely constitutes a true source of moral reflection.[118] With this methodology far more emphasis will be given to the emotional and socio-economic situation in which a woman finds herself. A decision will not be based solely on biological evidence or belief, but rather within the interlocking web of relationships which are normal for women's lives as they are for most people.

It is evident that the experience of women who have had or

who contemplate abortions should be a legitimate source for moral reflection. However, a methodology which is based primarily on the interweaving of relationships could easily develop into relativism. Our experience demonstrates that, due to a variety of factors, relationships develop and change within the course of a person's life. Should the flexibility of relationships be used as the primary foundation of the moral reflection on abortion? While retaining its principles Catholic theology should endeavour to ensure that moral reflection takes seriously the context and the experience of women who make decisions regarding abortion.

Another group of theologians has attempted to move away from the rigid interpretation of the 'double effect theory'. They also emphasise the important distinction that has to be drawn between 'morality' and 'pastoral care or practice'. Bernard Häring writes that moral theology operates on a level 'where questions are raised about general rules or considerations that would justify a particular moral judgment'.[119] A moral statement is thus an abstract statement, not in the sense that it has nothing to do with real life or with particular decisions, but in the sense that it abstracts or rescinds from the ability of this or that person to understand it and live it. Pastoral care (and pastoral statements), by contrast, looks to the art of the possible. It deals with the individual—where this person is in terms of his or her strengths, perceptions, biography, circumstances (financial, medical, educational, familial, psychological). Although pastoral care attempts to expand perspectives and maximise strengths, it recognises at times the limits of these attempts.[120]

With regard to situations in which the life of the mother and the fetus conflict it is proposed that conflict situations cannot be solved merely by the physical structure and causality of the act. Rather the human values involved in taking of life must be seen as a reluctant necessity. However, 'in the case of abortion there can arise circumstances in which the abortion is justified for preserving the life of the mother or for some other important value commensurate with life even though the action itself aims at abortion as a means to an end'.[121]

Bernard Häring and Franz Boeckle reason that in these situations it is not a matter of preferring either the life of the mother to the child or the child to the mother, but a choice between the life that can be saved and the life that cannot. In these instances the sole choice is to let both die or save the life of the mother. In such an intervention the child is already deprived of any chance to be kept alive, and its life is shortened by only a brief period. Boeckle goes on to state that in cases of vital conflict it is the medical institutions which determine the interruption of pregnancy. Beyond this case he does not see any plausible reasons that could morally justify an interruption of pregnancy.[122] It follows that with this direct intervention the life of the mother is saved, and that the potential for bearing future children is also preserved. In a further development of this argumentation, Häring considered situations in which the continuation of pregnancy, although not life threatening, would cause 'grave damage' to the mother. He considers the opinion probable of those who justify the removal of a fetus that surely cannot survive, when the action is taken in order to prevent grave damage to the mother. For instance, 'an anencephalic fetus not only cannot develop into a conscious human life but cannot even survive. To remove it in order to spare great damage to the mother is truly therapeutic while no injustice is done to the life of this fetus already doomed to death.'[123] Häring states that traditional moral theology would have called this intervention an 'indirect abortion'. He does not elaborate on the meaning of 'grave damage', but in the context of the case cited it would seem to mean the grave emotional damage a woman could suffer knowing that her child would die within days of birth. There is a danger that 'grave damage' could be more broadly interpreted to apply to the detection with pre-natal diagnosis of a severe disease. Häring is quick to point out that therapeutic abortion is quite different from genetic indicators whose detection occurs with pre-natal diagnosis. In cases like this, he argues, the fetus and not the mother is the patient. Killing the patient is no therapy whatsoever.

In addressing the pastoral situation of rape, Häring says that it is morally permissible to cleanse away the sperm, which is considered to be an extension of the initial act of aggression. Abortion is not allowed if conception has already taken place. It cannot be concluded that the fetus, which would not have been formed except for the presence of the 'aggressive' sperm, is itself an 'aggressor'.[124] Nevertheless, it must be recognised that although the fetus is innocent, the woman likewise is innocent. Her feelings that this is not 'her' child which she is in justice required to bear, are understandable. He argues that the Catholic counsellor should try to motivate her to consider the child with love because of its subjective innocence, and to bring it to term. If, owing to the psychological effects of her traumatic experience, she is utterly unable to accept this counsel, it is possible that she should be left in 'invincible ignorance'. 'Invincible ignorance', a traditional term in Catholic theology, refers to the existential wholeness of the person, the overall inability to cope with a certain moral imperative. This inability can exist not only with regard to the highest ideals of the Gospel, but also with regard to the particular prohibited norm. On this basis Häring concludes that the counsellor should not pursue the question once it has become evident that the woman could not bear the burden of pregnancy, nor bear the burden of a clear appeal not to abort.[125]

It is evident that both Boeckle and Häring attempt to broaden the traditional interpretation of 'indirect abortion'. Their cautious approach ensures that primarily only physically life-threatening conditions are addressed. However, what of the situation of a pregnant woman who threatens suicide because of her pregnancy? Does not this threat fall into the category of a vital conflict between the life of the mother and that of the child? There is a fear that, due to the difficulty of gauging the gravity of suicidal intentionality, any move in this direction will open the way for the justification of direct abortion in almost any circumstance. However, this is to disregard the gravity of the very real distress some women feel when confronted with an unwanted pregnancy and how these feelings of absolute hopelessness can lead to the desire to end their lives. It could be argued that this distress is a normal reaction in someone faced with an unwanted pregnancy and that these feelings will pass given appropriate support and counselling. But what of the cases in which support and therapy do not work and a very real likelihood exists that the woman will attempt to take her own life? I think it could be probable to argue that in cases of this type a truly physical life-threatening situation has arisen and that abortion could be considered therapeutic and indirect. In this instance it is not a matter of preferring either the life of the mother to the child or the child to the mother, but a choice between the life that can be saved and the life that cannot.

As can be seen from papal teaching and Catholic theology there has been a consistency in the condemnation of direct abortion. But moral absolutism of this type can be a liability as well as a strength. The distance between absolutist pronouncements and the pastoral situation can become unbridgeable. Where this occurs the voice of idealism can be rejected totally. Catholic theology needs to keep open the lines of dialogue with the other Christian denominations who have also confronted this issue. Polarisation of positions is not the way forward. Rather an honest dialogue which sets out to apply Christian ideals in the pastoral situation can be both theologically enriching and responsive to the very real pastoral needs of people.

PROTESTANT THEOLOGICAL TEACHING ON THE MORALITY OF ABORTION

Many Christian thinkers and in fact several Christian churches regard abortion under certain circumstances as licit and moral. In some cases, for certain Protestant theologians, abortion could even be a duty. The position of these thinkers and the teachings of their churches are honestly held beliefs and therefore need to be taken seriously by all sincere Christians.

The question to be raised is why, within the Christian tradition, two divergent beliefs can be arrived at from the same sources? The reason for this is two diverse world views. The traditional Catholic position, with roots in the ancient past, was dominated by a particular concept of nature. Here sexuality and procreation were understood as being part of nature, watched over by divine providence. Sexuality is, therefore, a biological function directed towards procreation of the human race. While there is pleasure attached to sexuality, it is orientated by its very nature to the begetting of children. It is not for parents to choose the number of children. To practise birth control or to provoke abortion is an interference with the order of nature and hence gravely sinful. From this perspective, abortion is seen among the sins against nature, touching on the procreative process of human life.

Due to a reaction, in recent years, by many Catholics to the official teaching on birth control, new and stronger arguments against abortion have become necessary. These arguments now centre around the destruction of fetal life which is believed to be fully human. What was condemned and abhorred in the past as a sin against the order of nature is now described as the taking of innocent life or murder.

The more liberal position on abortion, adopted by some Protestant churches, fits into a world picture that is dominated by the concept of history. According to this belief people do not enter into their destiny by conforming to a given order of nature, but by assuming responsibility for themselves and their environment and by creating their own future. God's providence is therefore not a guidance from above, but a gracious action with human life, freeing and enabling people to expand the area of their own responsibility. Sexuality, conception and procreation, while grounded in biology, belong properly to the sphere of history. Humans are called on by God to assume responsibility for them. Sexuality is not just perceived under the biological aspect: it is a wider human reality, with deep meaning and power, and men and women are summoned to integrate the sexual dimension into their lives in a healing, joyful and reconciling manner. The number of children is the responsibility of the parents. God's providence is believed to be operative through the grace-sustained free choice of mother and father. Abortion is, therefore, an extreme interference in the life process, prompted by people's responsibility for the future, which to many theologians seems justified, at least under certain conditions. They argue that it is the parents' responsibility to take the decision, in cases of emergency, to interrupt a pregnancy with a clinical intervention. It is a view dominated by people's increasing responsibility for the future, for the number of children born and for the kinds of lives these children will have, that explains how theologians and Christian churches can come to acknowledge abortion as a moral choice in extreme cases.[126]

It is not possible to give a comprehensive survey of the teachings of all the Protestant churches on abortion. I, therefore, intend to appraise only four. They represent distinctive traditions within Protestantism and cover most of the arguments used by the Protestant community. A similar methodology will be applied when discussing the various theological arguments advanced by several theologians.

Protestant fundamentalism in the USA
Fundamentalism in the United States of America is actually a loose federation of independent churches representing approximately thirty million people. Its description cannot be confined to merely doctrinal questions, but must also include its spirit or style. The doctrinal foundations were set forth in *The Fundamentals* published between 1910 and 1915. Central among them is the notion of biblical inerrancy and infallibility, which is the current test for orthodox belief and for Christian fellowship in this group. However, the spirit of fundamentalism is even more determinative of the nature of the movement. It is a religious mentality which is characterised by an arrogance that considers itself normative in all matters of theology and morality. Fundamentalists zealously perceive themselves as God's chosen agents for the salvation of the world.[127]

Their position on abortion hinges on the providence of God and the view that the fetus is a human person from conception. God is, therefore, the cause of and controller of all natural processes. This view is essential to their absolutist stance against abortion. Not only is the conceptus regarded as of equal value and personhood with the woman, but conception is the consequence of an act of God. 'What, therefore, God hath joined together, let no person put asunder', is, for fundamentalists, a biblical principle applicable to the abortion debate. What is at stake in the fundamentalist's position is a Calvinist stress on the sovereignty of God. This stress combines theological notions of power and activity of God with a type of natural law, similar to but without the sophistication of the natural law theory in Roman Catholic thought. The 'causal connection between sexual intercourse and conception . . . is simply the means whereby God, the first cause of all things, gives his blessing.'[128] In other words, however it happens in nature is the way God does it.[129]

Fundamentalists usually agree that the fetus may be terminated when the life of the woman is at stake. In such a case, it is a life for a life (Ex. 21:23).[130] They also recognise that the command forbidding killing in the Old Testament is not an absolute one. However, they draw back from applying this to abortion for at least two reasons. First, no injunction permitting abortion appears in the Bible. Second, fundamentalists argue that the fetus is innocent human life and thus to be protected.[131]

The real reason, however, behind their opposition to abortion is the belief that abortion violates an absolute moral rule based on the assumption that the fetus is a human being from the moment of conception. By using certain texts such as Exodus 21:22–5[132] they attempt to demonstrate that there is biblical evidence to support their claim that the fetus is a human being and that abortion is murder and thus should be legally forbidden.

Some Protestant churches in the United Kingdom

The proposed legislation for abortion in 1967 sparked off a heated debate within the various churches in the United Kingdom. This debate was to continue after legislation was passed making abortion, in certain circumstances, legal. It might prove helpful to give a brief summary of present British abortion legislation. It is difficult to assess the impact of this legislation on the world; but we do know that it was used as the basis for a liberalisation of abortion legislation in many parts of the world. Within the United States of America it was to influence fundamentally the debate which led to the liberalisation of American abortion law by the Supreme Court in 1973.[133]

The *1967 Abortion Act*, introduced by Mr David Steele MP as a private members bill, permits an abortion to be legally carried out on one or more of the following grounds:

1   The continuance of the pregnancy would involve risk to the life of the pregnant woman greater than if the pregnancy were terminated;

2   The continuance of pregnancy would involve risk of injury to the physical or mental health of the pregnant woman greater than if the pregnancy were terminated;

3   The continuance of the pregnancy would involve risk or injury to the physical or mental health of an existing child(ren) in the family of the pregnant woman greater than if the pregnancy were terminated;

4   There is a substantial risk if the child were born it would suffer from such physical or mental abnormalities as to be seriously handicapped.

    Or in an emergency, two grounds taken from the *1929 Infant Life (Preservation) Act*:

5   To save the life of the pregnant woman;

6   To prevent grave permanent injury to the physical or mental health of the pregnant woman.

The 1967 Act did not define an upper limit for the time in pregnancy when the abortion may be carried out. This was determined by the 1929 Act which stated that 28 weeks was when a child could be born alive.

Government figures[134] show that in 1976, ground 2 of the 1967 Act accounted for 83.5% of all stated grounds for abortion in England and Wales, and in 1989 this had risen to 88.6%. The risk of handicap in the baby, ground 4 of the 1967 Act, accounted for 1.3% and 1% in those years respectively.

With effect from 1 April 1991 the law on abortion was changed as a result of the decision of both Houses of Parliament on free votes to add a clause to the *Human Fertilisation and Embryology Bill*. This amended the 1967 Act as follows:

a   It inserts a 24-week time limit for abortions in grounds 2 and 3;

b   It provides that ground 1 and ground 4 will be without time limit;

c   It introduces a new ground for abortion (without time limit) to prevent grave permanent injury to the physical or mental health of the pregnant woman. (this wording appears as ground 6 in relation to emergency abortion in the 1967 Act);

d   It allows account to be taken of the pregnant woman's actual or reasonably foreseeable environment in cases of termination on the new ground set out in (c) above;

e   It permits the Secretary of State to authorise the use of specified abortifacient drugs, if they are in future licensed and marketed in Britain, in places other than an NHS hospital or an approved nursing home;

f   It makes clear that selective reduction of a pregnancy (termination of one or more, but not all, fetuses in a multiple pregnancy) may be performed if the requirements of the Abortion Act are fulfilled, but not otherwise;

g   It provides that in England and Wales abortions under the Abortion Act 1967 will no longer be governed by the 28-week presumption of fetal viability in the Infant Life (Preservation) Act. (The 1929 Act has never applied in Scotland).

In respect of abortions performed after 24 weeks there will be no change in the previous arrangements whereby NHS hospitals are the only places where such abortions may be carried out.

Both the 1967 Act and the Amended 1991 Act are fully comprehensive and allow abortion not only to preserve the physical health of the mother, but also permit abortions for 'social reasons'. These 'social reasons' can be found in sections 2 and 3 of the 1967 Act and c and d of the 1991 Amendment. In these clauses provision is made not just for the impact of pregnancy on the mental health of the woman but also its effect on her family. Consideration is also given to the woman's actual and foreseeable environment. By permitting the family and environment to become part of the moral consideration the law has ensured that social reasons such as marital status, employment prospects, housing facilities and family size are now all to be taken into consideration. The Lane Committee found that certain medical practitioners advised abortions in an attempt to address social problems such as housing, employment and single parenthood. It was this broadening of the justification of abortion which was to cause the various churches the greatest theological difficulties.

The Church of Scotland

The development of the theological teaching on abortion in the Church of Scotland is underpinned by a statement of the General Assembly in 1966 which states that: 'We cannot assert too strongly that the inviolability of the fetus is one of the fundamentals and its right to life must be strongly defended.'[135] This understanding allowed the Board's 1985 report to ground its opposition to abortion on the following principles. First it invoked the biblical teaching to demonstrate that the unborn child should be regarded as bearing the divine image and that Jesus Christ in his conception took upon himself manhood in utero. The report also invoked the 'unbroken tradition' of the Christian Church's antipathy to abortion. Finally in referring to the discoveries of modern genetics and embryology it argues that these 'confirm us in our belief that the foetus is an independent being, a tiny member of our species'.[136] In the light of this declaration, the Board were extremely critical of the 1967 Abortion Act and especially of its practical application. They went on to conclude that due to 'our belief in the sanctity of all human life we are convinced that the inviolability of the foetus can be brought into question only in the case of risk to maternal life and when all alternatives have been exhausted'.[137]

This position did not win unqualified support within the Church of Scotland and many of their theologians dissociated themselves from this decision.[138] Much of the opposition came from those who interpreted it as putting rape victims in a practically intolerable position. An ongoing debate ensued, mainly concerned with what approach should be taken towards 'cases of special difficulty' such as fetal abnormality, pregnancy through rape, or other such reasons. However, it was agreed that 'in the great majority of cases, abortion has no moral justification and represents the unwarranted destruction of human life that is made in the image of God'.[139] In the area of 'cases of special difficulty' opinion was divided. Some held to the 1985 belief that abortion was permissible only if the mother's life was in grave risk, while others supported the 1986 General Assembly view that the criteria for abortion be extended to include not only a 'serious risk to the life of the mother', but also a 'grave injury to the health, whether physical or mental, of the pregnant woman'. This view recognised the sanctity of life as one of the fundamental principles but also recognised that, in particular circumstances, the principle of relief of suffering may also justify the use of abortion. Supporters of this view also advocated the inclusion of another clause in the 1967 Act which justified abortion on the grounds of severe physical or mental handicap of the fetus.[140]

The Church of Scotland, therefore, recognised the differences within the church and felt that they had no alternative but to acknowledge these differences and to present them in such a way that all concerned might be helped to choose wisely and lovingly and to discover the will of God for themselves.[141]

The Church of England
In 1965 the Church of England Board for Social Responsibility published *Abortion, An Ethical Discussion* as the Anglican contribution to the debate which led to the 1967 Abortion Act. While accepting that not all Anglicans would agree with its position it nevertheless became the cornerstone of the Church of England's official position dealing specifically with abortion. It began by acknowledging that the fetus, as potential human life, has a significance which must not be overlooked, minimised or denied. However, the problem of abortion is centred on weighing the claims of the mother against the claims of the fetus and vice versa, when they conflict. The Board recognised the importance that neither the mother nor the fetus be thought of in isolation from the family group within which they exist. It goes on to argue that in certain circumstances abortion can be

justified. This would be when, at the request of the mother and after extensive consultation, it could be 'reasonably established that there was a threat to the mother's life or well-being, and hence inescapably to her health, if she were obliged to carry the child to term and give it birth'. However, the Board does point out that this decision by the mother must be taken within the context of her own life and well-being and the life and well-being of her family. It goes on to mention two possible grounds for abortion: the risk of a defective or deformed child and cases of incest or rape. Nevertheless, it qualifies this by arguing that the decision to abort should be determined by the effect the pregnancy will have on the mother and not the possibility of deformity itself, nor simply the fact of the act of incest or rape.[142]

Some years later the General Synod, sharing 'the widespread anxiety being felt in the country over the working of the Abortion Act 1967, passed resolutions in February 1974, July 1975 and November 1979 in favour of reforming the current law in order to correct the "manifest abuses" which were taking place under it'. Dr John Habgood pointed out that the safeguards and assurances given when the 1967 Act was passed have to a considerable extent been ignored. He felt that 'abortion has now become a live option for anybody who is pregnant. This does not imply that everyone who is facing an unwanted pregnancy automatically attempts to procure an abortion. But because abortion is now on the agenda, the climate of opinion in which such a pregnancy must be faced has radically altered.'[143]

In 1980 the Roman Catholic Archbishops of Great Britain issued an absolutist condemnation of current practices in Britain. The Board for Social Responsibility responded by stating that abortion is a 'great moral evil'. Nevertheless they recognised that circumstances exist where the character or location of the pregnancy render the fetus a serious threat to the life or health of the mother. In these circumstances the mother 'would be entitled to seek protection against the threat to her life and health which the fetal life represented'. If a choice had to be made between the life of the mother and the continuation of the pregnancy, precedence should be given to the mother's interests. However, such a choice would only arise 'if no less drastic remedy for the ill existed'. The Board goes on to point out that in European society with advanced facilities for pre-natal diagnosis and care such situations are highly exceptional. They recognise that women who resort to abortion today are encouraged for very different reasons, reasons which frequently highlight seriously unsatisfactory personal or family circumstances such as family size, single parenthood and the socio-economic factors of housing and employment. These circumstances, the Board argues, cannot morally justify the extreme step of abortion.[144]

At successive Synods resolutions were passed for the reform of the law on abortion. In February 1990 the Board once again examined the issue of abortion. It recognised the 'deep differences of judgment concerning abortion' which exist within the Church of England and other British churches. From the Christian point of view, the debate centres on the relative degrees of protection to be given to the fetus, mother and family. The first view stresses the sanctity of each life from its beginning and is committed to the right of the embryo to total protection. The second emphasises the status of the embryo as part of its mother, and calls for compassion towards the mother when a pregnancy is unwanted and recognises the right of the woman, sometimes or even always, to opt for abortion. The Board stresses that whatever point of view is adopted, it needs to be recognised that the possibility of abortion always arises from within a particular social and cultural setting, and is the creation of that setting.[145]

An important contribution to the discussion on abortion is the Board's recognition that Christians can be conscientiously divided on the morality of termination. It goes on to argue that the two positions outlined are held with deep conviction by their protagonists, and both claim scriptural support. Mindful that these positions could lead to deadlock they raise the question of whether this polarisation is inevitable or whether the elements of truth in both approaches can be affirmed. In an attempt to bring the two positions to a common understanding the Board begins by arguing that the Church is a body of people committed to seeking the will of God and to sharing the love of God. They affirm that every human life, created in the divine image, is unique and designed for loving relationships. Therefore, they believe that abortion is an evil because it denies this truth, and that abortion on demand would be a very great evil. However, the Board goes on to state that they believe that to withhold compassion is also evil, and in circumstances of extreme distress or need, a very great evil. 'To decide which is the lesser of the two can mean genuine dilemma and pain which should not be minimised, but Christians need to face frankly the fact that in an imperfect world the "right" choice is sometimes the acceptance of the lesser of two evils.'[146]

It is evident from the vigorous debate that has gone on within the Church of England that it believes: first, that all human life, including life developing in the womb, is to be protected; second, that it is extremely concerned about the large number of abortions being carried out under the current legislation; and third, recognises that there are situations in which abortion can be justified. The interpretation of these situations can differ within the Church of England. Some theologians would limit abortions only to life-threatening situations, while others would permit them for emotional or socio-economic reasons. However, what becomes evident in the Church of England's understanding of this issue is the desire to find a course of action which might not be perfect, but at least responds to the circumstances in which people find themselves. Abortion is an evil, but it may, in some circumstances, be the lesser of two evils.

The Methodist Church

In 1976 the Methodist Church at their National Conference adopted a formal statement on abortion which was to colour future theological reflection. This statement laid down the theological principles which were to guide their judgments on abortion. The Conference began by affirming the Christian belief that the person is a creature of God, made in the divine image, and that human life, though marred, has eternal as well as physical and material dimensions. Recognising that the fetus is part of the continuum of human existence, the Conference argued that future study was necessary to determine the extent to which the fetus is a person. In their discussion of this point they assert that persons are created for relationships with God and with other people. Christians must reflect in human relationships their response to God's love. They point out that although the fetus possesses a degree of individual identity, it lacks independence and the ability to respond to relationships. Therefore in considering the matter of abortion, the Christian asks 'what person, or beings who are properly to be treated wholly or in part as persons, are involved, and how they will be affected by a decision to permit or forbid abortion'.[147]

The statement goes on to remind Christians of their duty to stand by people in times of crisis and help them make responsible decisions. It also warns that human judgments may be impaired by sin and that abortion decisions may be made 'in a context of selfishness, carelessness or exploitation'.[148] It then proceeds to analyse the issues involved. They point to the two views current within the Methodist Church. The first stresses the value and importance of all forms of human life by asserting that the fetus has an inviolable right to life and that there must be no external interference with the process which will lead to the birth of a living human being. The second emphasises the interests of the mother. The fetus is totally dependent on her for at least the first twenty weeks of pregnancy and, it is therefore argued, she has a total right to decide whether or not to continue the pregnancy. It is further argued that a child has the right to be born healthy and wanted. Both views, the Conference recognises, make points of real value. On the one hand, the significance of human life should not be diminished, while on the other hand, abortion is unique because of the total physical dependence of the fetus on the mother, to whose life, capacities or existing responsibilities, the fetus may pose a threat of which she is acutely aware. They argue that it is also necessary to face this stark conflict of interests and to acknowledge that others are also involved—the father, the existing children of the family, the extended family, and society in general. The Conference, therefore, argues that 'there is never any moment from conception onwards when the fetus totally lacks human significance—a fact which may be overlooked in the pressure for abortion on demand'. However the degree of this significance manifestly increases. At the very least, they stress, no pregnancy should be aborted after the point when the aborted fetus has reached viability.[149]

The Methodist position insists on respect for the embryo but it maintains that this respect should be in keeping with the embryo's developing human status. It sees the achievement of the human dignity of the embryo as a gradual process and does not identify any one stage of the process as completely determinative.[150]

With this theological foundation they were now able to address the many difficult questions posed by the pastoral situation. In the case of a pregnancy that threatens the physical health of the mother they argue that an abortion may in these circumstances be the right course of action. This is based on the assumption that the life of the adult woman is of greater significance than that of the unborn.[151] They then go on to address the far more complex and common issue of abortion for 'social reasons'. Can the termination of a pregnancy which does not directly threaten the health of the mother ever be morally justified? Before a decision can be made, they maintain, a number of considerations need to be taken into account. While stressing that abortion must not be viewed as a solution to social problems they nevertheless recognise that not all abortions for 'social reasons' are necessarily 'wrong'. They point out that there are social circumstances where the death of the fetus is a lesser evil than the consequent suffering of those involved if it is allowed to be born. For example, a child conceived as a result of rape or incest may be utterly repugnant to the mother, thus making bonding impossible. Or a child born with severe handicap may attract all the emotional energy of the mother, leaving siblings deprived, and if later institutional care is needed for the handicapped child, parents may experience great stress and sense of failure.

The issue of the quality of life not just of the family, but also of the baby must be considered. The whole notion of 'quality of life' is a complex one. Many of the couples who find themselves in the situation of knowing that the mother is carrying an abnormal fetus will already have a child who has or is suffering from the disease. They will know that 'quality of life' is not something that is on a constant level. Suffering for the individual and stress for the family will be far worse at times than others. Prospective parents with little knowledge of what bringing up a diseased or handicapped child could mean will need to be provided with as much information as possible before they can be expected to make a decision.

Another issue that may well become more common in the future is the problem when a mother is carrying the human immunodeficiency virus (i.e. is HIV-positive) or has the symptoms of AIDS. It is known that the virus can be transferred to the fetus. In addition to the problem of the quality of life for the mother and baby (including the attitude of society to them) there is the risk of spreading the infection further.

Although in normal circumstances human life is to be valued in its own right, there are occasions when it is acceptable to abort the unborn human in order to minimise suffering if this is what the parents, having been fully informed and supported, feel is right. It is not easy to give hard and fast rules as to when this is the case, but an example might be the particularly distressing disease affecting the haemoglobin, Bart's hydrops syndrome.[152]

The Methodist Church while considering the expanding science of pre-natal diagnosis argues that Christians must provide a clear expression of the value of all human beings before God so that a framework is established to think through the moral implications of the use to which the new knowledge gained may be put.[153]

PROTESTANT THEOLOGIANS

The great German Protestant theologian Karl Barth addresses the question of abortion by pointing out that 'there can be no doubt that the abstract prohibition which was pronounced in the past, and which is still the only contribution of Roman Catholicism in this matter, is far too forbidding and sterile to promise any effective help'.[154] When considering abortion Barth encourages a cautious view. The Christian presumption must always tend to be 'No' in matters of abortion. However he goes on to point out that human life, and therefore the life of the unborn is not an absolute. It cannot claim to be preserved in all circumstances, whether in relation to God or other persons, i.e., in this case to the mother, father, doctor, or others involved.[155] He therefore argues that there are exceptional cases. 'Let us be quite frank and say that there are situations in which the killing of germinating life does not constitute murder but is in fact commanded.'[156] He points out that such exceptions will nevertheless be very rare. Barth, in other articles on the topic, would appear to allow abortion only when the life of the mother was threatened.[157]

The late Professor Paul Ramsey of Princeton, an influential Protestant theologian, was a strong opponent of abortion. Writing before 'Roe v. Wade' (1973)[158] was decided, he insisted that even the use of intrauterine contraceptive devices, which prevent the implantation of a fertilised egg, was sinful, and he suggested that all young girls be given German measles deliberately to immunise them from that disease so that it would not be necessary to abort any fetuses damaged because a woman contracted the disease in pregnancy. But Ramsey made plain that his strong opinions were based not on the assumption of fetal personhood or rights, but on the principle of the 'sanctity of human life'. A person must respect his or her own life and the lives of others not only because life is grounded in God, but, equally important, because God has given a person life as a value to be held in trust and used according to God's will. 'From this point of view,' he said,

it is relatively unimportant to say exactly when among the products of human generation we are dealing with an organism that is human and when we are dealing with organic life that is not human. . . . A man's dignity is an overflow from God's dealings with him, and not primarily an anticipation of anything he will ever be by himself alone. . . . The Lord did not set his love upon you, nor choose you because you were already intrinsically more than a blob of tissues in the uterus.[159]

Ramsey argued that it is respect for God's creative choice and love of humanity, not any rights of a 'blob of tissue in the uterus' that makes abortion sinful.[160]

Dr James Wood Jr, executive director of the Baptist Joint Committee on Public Affairs, reports that Baptists are divided about abortion and that there is no official Baptist position. In 1976 the Southern Baptist Convention in the United States rejected any 'discriminate attitude toward abortion, as contrary to biblical views' but refused to adopt a submitted resolution that declared, 'Every decision for an abortion, for whatever reason, must necessarily involve the decision to terminate the life of an innocent human being.' Dr Wood said that in his own opinion, sound Baptist faith condemned abortion for frivolous reasons but recognised it as permissible when pregnancy was involuntary (including pregnancies of very young girls not of an age to consent and of women whose contraceptive devices had failed), cases of fetal deformity, and cases where significant family reasons argued against pregnancy.[161]

The Revd John Wagoman, a Methodist minister, argued that 'it is a common view among Protestant theologians, and to some extent among other religious bodies, that human personhood—in the sense in which the person receives its maximum value in relation to the Christian faith—does not exist in the earlier stages of pregnancy . . . there is not a fully human person until that stage in development where someone has begun to have experience of reality.' 'In bringing new life into the world human beings must be sure that the conditions into which the new life is being born will sustain that life in accordance with God's intention for the life to be fulfilled.' A pregnant woman 'responding out of faith and love of God to the love which God has provided to human beings' might decide to have an abortion when the new life would be unlikely to receive the nurture necessary for human fulfilment, either because she is herself only a teenager, for example, or because she is close to menopause or because the existence of a new child would make life much harder for the existing family.[162]

James Gustafson's approach is considered by many to be the most influential of Protestant approaches. He begins by stating three principles and three exceptions:

1   Life is to be preserved rather than destroyed.
2   Those who cannot assert their own rights to life are especially to be protected.
3   There are exceptions to these rules.

Possible exceptions are:

a   'medical indications' that make therapeutic abortion morally viable.
b   the pregnancy has occurred as a result of sexual crime. (I would grant this as a viable possible exception in every instance . . . if the woman herself was convinced that it was right. If the woman sees the exception as valid, she has a right to more than a potentially legal justification for her decision; as a person she has the right to understand why it is an exception in her dreadful plight.)
c   the social and emotional conditions do not appear to be beneficial for the well-being of the mother and the child. (In particular circumstances, this may appear to be justification, but I would not resort to it until possibilities for financial, social, and spiritual help have been explored.)[163]

What is crucially important to Gustafson is compassion for the woman involved, and her ability to make a human decision grounded in freedom of choice. Nevertheless, seeing the tragedy of abortion, he, with an allusion to war, argues that as the morally conscientious soldier fighting in a particular war is convinced that life can and ought to be taken, 'justly' but also 'mournfully',[164] so the moralist can be convinced that the life of the defenceless fetus can be taken, less justly, but more mournfully.[165]

Stanley Hauerwas approaches the morality of abortion from a different viewpoint. He begins by examining three questions relating to abortion: When does life begin? When may life be taken legitimately? What does the agent understand to be happening? Having answered the first two in classical terms he turns to the third question. He contends that there is more in an agent's deliberation and decision that are morally important than in the spectator's judgment. This 'more' is the agent's perspective. To illustrate how this perspective works he takes a situation presented by the Protestant theologian, James Gustafson—a very tragic instance of pregnancy resulting from multiple rape in a situation of poverty, illness and lack of employment. Gustafson argues that because the pregnancy resulted from a sex crime and the social and emotional considerations for the well-being of the mother and child are not advantageous, the abortion would be morally justified.

Hauerwas defends Gustafson's approach, not on the basis that abortion is a good thing, but rather because 'abortion is morally justified under an ethical perspective that tries to pull as much good as possible from the situation'. It might be different if societal conditions and the woman's biography favoured and supported carrying the pregnancy to term. Hauerwas claims that moral choices do not occur in ideal conditions where right and wrong are apparent, but rather the right must be wrenched from less than ideal alternatives.[166]

An ordained minister and consultant gynaecologist, R. F. Gardner justifies abortion by arguing that the fetus does not possess a soul, and therefore we are not considering the destruction of a human life destined for eternity. He suggests that it is when the child takes his or her first breath that the soul enters the body.[167] Three 'scientific pointers' are offered to support this thesis. First, the question of identical twins. At some point after conception, and sometimes even after implantation, the embryo divides into two. 'Unless', writes Gardner, 'we are to agree with the suggestion that the soul splits likewise we are driven to conclude that in some cases at least its infusion is not before the fourth week of intrauterine life.'[168] Second, he draws attention to the phenomenon of fetal 'wastage' whereby 'anything up to half of all conceptions end in spontaneous miscarriages, usually very early on'.[169] He considers it inconceivable that God should fill his heaven with these young lives, and concludes that it is evidence of the absence of 'spiritual status' on the part of the fetus. Third,

to suggest that embryos cultured *in vitro* and experimented upon
and then disposed of possess a soul would be to trivialise the
'meaning of the soul'.

Having disposed of the 'spiritual status' of the fetus Gardner
advances his own grounds for justifying abortion. His starting-
point is Christian compassion. 'Real compassion', he suggests,
'involves taking into account medical and social factors.'[170] His
compassionate aim is not just to alleviate a woman's short-term
problem, but also to facilitate a better future life for her.
However, he does point out that for the Christian physician, it is
not just a matter of responding to a distressing situation but also
of trying to determine the will of God in that particular situation.
His discernment process for arriving at a decision appears to be
an examination of the physical, psychological, spiritual, social
and economic factors which impact on the life of his patient.

For these theologians, and those who agree with their ethics,
the defence of abortion generally operates on the principle of
denying to the fetus, at some stage or at all stages, the respect
due to full human life outside the womb.[171]

As can be observed from this brief survey of the views of
certain Christian churches all agree that the human embryo has
'value' and must be respected. The disagreement concerns what
precisely is the 'value' of the human embryo. One view,
represented explicitly by the Roman Catholic Church, states that
it has exactly the same value as any other human being. Another
view, represented by a strong body of opinion in the Church of
England, asserts that its value, prior to individuation
(consciousness), is less than that of a human being in the proper
sense of the word. A third view, represented by the Methodist
Conference, would argue that its value depends on its stage of
development: thus a progressively increasing value. The Baptist
Union seems to favour a similar position, as does the Church in
Wales and the Free Churches.[172]

The implications of these approaches for abortion are quite
clear. When the value given to the embryo is exactly the same as
that given to any other human being, then the good of the
embryo cannot be directly sacrificed for the good of any other

human beings involved. This view, therefore rules out every act of direct abortion. When full human value is given to the embryo only after the point of definitive individuation has been reached, then prior to that moment the good of the embryo takes second place when it is in conflict with full human beings. If the human embryo is considered to have less-than-fully-human but progressively increasing value up to the time of birth, then respect for full human dignity would justify abortion right through the whole of pregnancy. According to this view, it would be a violation of human dignity to subordinate the good of a human being to that of a being, despite its intrinsic value, which is not fully human. The reasons for abortion, however, would need to increase in gravity in proportion to the lateness of the pregnancy.[173]

It also emerges from certain Protestant theologians that the emotional and environmental context of pregnancy needs to be seriously considered. The Christian virtue of compassion is often invoked as a justifiable response to a distressing situation. Admittedly these are very serious factors which need to be included in the course of moral decision-making. But they presuppose a maturity of faith and the ability to arrive at clear and informed conscience decisions. If this maturity is not evident moral decision-making could easily become purely relative. However, owing to these diverse views on the morality of abortion numerous governments have legislated for abortion where the fetus is perceived to be a direct threat to the life of the mother, or where the fetus is seen to endanger the 'health' of the mother. 'Health' in this sense can have a very broad interpretation depending on how it is defined in various legal traditions. Catholics, Häring advises, although they might not find the reasons concerning a broad definition of health convincing, should not oppose the legislation of a pluralistic state that leaves freedom in these cases to the physicians and the mothers to decide according to their conscience.[174]

2

MORAL QUESTIONS POSED
BY IN VITRO FERTILISATION AND
EMBRYO EXPERIMENTATION

The birth of Louise Brown in 1978, the first test-tube baby, brought into the public domain the science of in vitro fertilisation and its related areas. This initiated a moral debate on reproduction-aiding techniques such as artificial insemination, surrogate motherhood and in vitro fertilisation. The question of experimentation on the early embryo also became an issue of moral enquiry. Underlying the moral debate on experimentation and reproduction-aiding technologies is the moral status of the embryo. What do people believe the embryo to be? Is it a full human being with potential or a potential human being? How this question is answered will determine the direction of future aided reproduction procedures and the important issue of embryo experimentation. The Christian churches have taken these questions extremely seriously and have responded with official statements. Our task will be to examine the various procedures resorted to, the moral status of the embryo and how this affects experimentation. Finally we will examine the responses of the Christian churches to in vitro fertilisation and experimentation on the embryo.

SEXUAL REPRODUCTION

Unaided reproduction
It is apt that we begin with the biology and physiology of natural reproduction, that is, the conception of a child by a man and a woman through unaided and un-supplemented sexual intercourse and the subsequent biological process. Humans reproduce sexually, that is, through the union of two cells

(gametes): the egg (ovum; plural ova)[1] from the female and sperm from the male. These gametes carry the genetic code of the male and the female. In reproduction the egg and sperm combine to form a single cell from which a new individual develops. The genetic make-up of the new cell is a combination of the genes from the egg and the sperm.

Normally fertilisation takes place in a fallopian tube and generally occurs within 10 to 15 hours of ovulation. In fertilisation, a sperm penetrates the egg's jelly-like coat, the coat changes to prevent additional sperm from entering, and the egg undergoes one further cell division, allowing for the last stage of fertilisation, the union of genetic materials of the egg and sperm. The result, if all goes well, is a single cell containing in its nucleus the full human complement of 23 pairs of chromosomes,[2] half contributed by the sperm and half by the egg.

The fertilised egg is at first called a zygote. During the four or five days it takes to reach the uterus, the zygote undergoes several cell divisions. When it reaches the uterus, the mass of about 16 cells rearranges itself into a hollow ball of cells called a blastocyst. The cells in the blastocyst continue to divide until the outer layer of cells makes contact with the uterine lining and attaches to it in the process called implantation. Some of the cells of the blastocyst develop into the placenta and fetal membrane, and some develop into the fetus itself. Following implantation, additional connections are made between the mother and the embryo to ensure that sufficient nutrients are available for development. As the embryo grows, membranous structures project into the uterine wall and provide for attachment. The region of attachment is known as the placenta. A secondary membrane, the amnion, surrounds the embryo and provides the local environment in which the embryo grows. This extensive tissue system provides for the maintenance of the embryo during its continued division, differentiation and development throughout pregnancy.

A number of important stages or events in the development of the embryo should be noted:

- At the two- and four-cell stage each cell is totipotential; that is, separated cells retain the potential to form separate embryos, which could result in the birth of identical twins.
- By about day 14 to 15 a heap of cells, called the 'primitive streak', develops in the embryo. If two primitive streaks develop, then identical twins occur.
- Brain activity: primitive brain cells have been claimed to occur as early as the 40th day, though it is not clear how these electrical impulses relate to what we understand to be consciousness.
- Viability: the point at which the fetus can survive outside the womb. This point depends on the state of neonatal technology and presently occurs at around 24 weeks.
- Parturition: birth, usually around 40 weeks after conception.[3]

Reproduction relies upon a number of anatomical and hormonal systems, so it is not surprising that reproduction is not always successful. It has been estimated that even when sperm do reach the egg in natural reproduction, for every 100 eggs only 84 are fertilised, 69 implant, 42 survive the first week of pregnancy and 31 survive to birth. For many individuals even this proportion does not hold. The figure of 15% is widely cited as the incidence of infertility among couples in the United States of childbearing age.[4] Infertility also has been generally held to be on the rise. Both the 15% figure and the rising incidence of infertility have been disputed, but even on lower estimates 2.4 million couples were infertile, in the United States of America, in 1982, and a total of $1 billion was spent in 1987 by couples seeking professional help for infertility.[5]

Reproduction-aiding technologies

For millions of couples natural reproduction does not work. The conditions and living patterns of modern society have been cited as causing infertility. Environmental pollutants and day-to-day stress are commonly thought to be particularly at fault. The relatively new patterns of short and varied sexual encounters, resulting disease, the unforeseen side effects of extensive use of birth control methods, are also seen as being contributing factors. Perhaps most significant, couples today are choosing to start families later in life, even though the incidence of infertility increases with age, dramatically so for women after the age of 30. Physiologically, two leading causes of fertility disorder are hormone malfunction and anatomical abnormalities, congenital or acqual, such as occluded fallopian tubes or an enlarged blood vessel in a testis.[6]

In an effort to aid these couples with severe problems, alternatives to natural reproduction have been developed. Why are people, particularly women, prepared to engage in what are considered by many to be intrusive medical procedures to ensure conception and birth?

By and large the new technologies of aided-reproduction are a response to a definite felt need amongst people. Therefore to fully understand the debate concerning this area it would be helpful to examine, in itself, the reactions to infertility in men and women and why they go to often extreme measures to procreate. An understanding of these reactions should assist us in making clear and informed moral judgments on aided-reproduction procedures.

Most patients seem to go through a number of phases in dealing with the infertility crisis;[7] these stages may vary in length and often overlap. The first phase revolves around the narcissistic injury. Acknowledgment of an infertility problem, whether it is after six months, one year, or several years of attempting to achieve a pregnancy, is a tremendous blow. Infertile patients often feel damaged, defective, and 'bad'. This sense of 'badness' may not remain confined to reproductive function alone, but may encompass sexual function and desirability, physical attractiveness, performance and productivity in other spheres as well.[8] Several female patients have described feeling like 'neuters', not belonging to any group classifiable as male or female, while male patients often refer to intercourse in these circumstances as 'shooting blanks'.[9] Concerns about sexual identity and sexual function are almost universal among infertile patients. In both men and women there is usually a significant diminution of sexual desire. The depression of both partners consequent to their unsuccessful efforts to achieve a pregnancy, the necessity for sexual relations on demand at specific times in the woman's cycle, and the concern about whether this time will be successful contribute heavily to the problems of sexual function commonly seen in infertile couples.[10] Sex is no longer a spontaneous, pleasurable activity; it is an assignment, a mission with a definable goal, i.e. pregnancy. Many try to be extra good to atone for whatever sins, real or imagined, they feel may have caused their infertility.[11] They may feel intense guilt, sometimes focused on a past event (e.g. an abortion), which may or may not be related to the current problem. Often their guilt is experienced in a diffuse way—guilt about oedipal wishes, guilt about masturbation and guilt about sexual fantasies of any kind.

Relations between partners often become strained and tense. The infertile spouse may fear actual or emotional abandonment by the other. The fertile partner may feel an obligation to maintain a front of loyalty, to disavow any disappointment or anger. There can also be jealousy of siblings which may extend to the entire female population. Many patients seriously restrict their lives and cut off old friendships in order to avoid confrontation with pregnant women or families with young babies. This isolation serves only to increase their sense of defectiveness.

Many patients see their infertility as a pronouncement of 'unfitness' for parenthood. They are disproportionately enraged by those who seem to take it for granted—e.g. people who abuse or neglect their children or those who favour abortion on demand. Some patients express more abstract fears about not being able to produce anything of value, accomplish anything of worth. During the tumult of the infertility treatment it is, in fact, more difficult to concentrate on studies or career.[12]

It is during this period that various aid-reproductive techniques are attempted. If these fail then patients often turn to adoption or, in cases of male infertility, artificial insemination by donor. Or they could come to terms with being childless and the grief and sense of failure this often involves. This may be especially difficult for those couples who have for many years focused their lives around the single-minded goal of pregnancy. For them the infertility work-up and treatment have become a substitute for a child, perhaps their only common interest or the only way in which they can demand or give each other emotional support. It may be difficult to wean such couples from their dependence on their infertility problems. For each individual and couple, the resolution of the problem is unique and is often determined by prior experiences of coping with disappointment and loss. Patients need to be assisted to establish an identity and meaning for life that does not include reproduction.[13]

In general reproductive-aiding techniques fall into two categories: those in which the roles of genetic, gestational and social parents remain as they are in natural reproduction; and those in which the provider of the sperm, egg or gestational functions is other than one of the social parents. The following methods describe briefly different forms of assisted reproduction and certain questions raised in relation to them.

Artificial insemination
There are two basic forms of artificial insemination: homologous artificial insemination (AIH) and artificial insemination by donor (AID).[14] In the first instance, the woman's husband is the source of the seminal fluid, whereas in the second instance an unknown male donor or a known male donor, possibly the husband's brother, is the source of the sperm and seminal fluid. With both procedures, the seminal fluid is placed into a syringe which is attached to a long cannula which is in turn placed against the external cervical canal. Inseminations are usually performed twice per cycle, usually just before and just after ovulation. Nearly three-fourths of patients, for whom this procedure is recommended, conceive if they continue therapy for one year.[15] If these attempts are unsuccessful after one year, donor sperm may be used with the IVF procedure with a reasonable success rate occurring after approximately six cycles.[16]

Surrogate motherhood

Society has tended to focus attention on the problems encountered if the surrogate mother conceives with sperm other than the recipient father's, if the mother does not wish to relinquish the child after delivery, and if the child born is abnormal. Normally the recipient father's sperm is used to inseminate artificially the surrogate mother who carries the pregnancy and who then gives the baby to the recipient couple. The surrogate mother is usually paid £6,500 to £10,000 with legal and medical fees also covered. The legality of this process appears to be in limbo in most countries.[17] Many independent and governmental studies actively discourage this procedure.[18]

In vitro fertilisation (IVF)

In vitro fertilisation (IVF)[19] is the procedure whereby so-called test-tube babies are conceived. Actually, in vitro simply means in glass, and IVF is the union of sperm and egg outside of the body—usually in a glass petri dish. Though it may sound simple, it is a complex and delicate procedure. Years of research and many failures preceded the first successful IVF birth, that is Louise Brown in 1978, under the care of Robert Edwards and Patrick Steptoe.

The technique of IVF varies somewhat, but normally the female undergoes controlled ovarian hyper-stimulation (is super ovulated) by using ovulating drugs. Ultra-sound monitoring is used to determine the ripening stage of the eggs. They are then retrieved just prior to expected ovulation. This traditionally has been accomplished by performing a laparoscopy under general anaesthesia, but recently it has been refined by using vaginal ultrasound for oocyte retrieval.[20] Sperm is collected by masturbation, washed and added to the eggs for incubation for 48 to 72 hours.

Development of the embryo outside the uterus is critically important to IVF. If the embryo is introduced into the uterus either too early or too late, implantation will not occur. While the embryo is incubating, the woman is given a progesterone injection, to prepare her uterus for implantation. Two days after fertilisation, the conceptus has developed to about eight cells. At this stage, it is ready to be placed in the uterus. Introduction into the uterus is achieved through a long catheter inserted through the vagina and cervix.

For reasons not yet fully understood, implantation seems to work best if several embryos are placed in the uterus; four appear to be the optimal number. When multiple embryos are introduced, usually only one implants and develops; the others are discharged from the woman's body. Occasionally, more than one embryo implants, and multiple births result.

Overall, success rates for IVF are not very high; even the best clinics claim not more than a 15 to 20% success rate, and many have no success. The cost per attempt is usually £2,000, and the total cost of treatment is several times that, with no assurance of success. Apart from the monetary costs, IVF can be an ordeal both psychologically and physically. Still, IVF has grown rapidly in popularity and approximately 15,000 IVF babies have been born worldwide. For many couples, IVF is the last chance, at the end of a long and trying struggle, to have a child who is biologically their own.[21]

GIFT (gamete intra fallopian transfer), TOT (tubal ovum transfer) and LTOT (lower tubal ovum transfer)

Due to opposition to IVF, particularly by the Roman Catholic Church, two other types of procedure have been developed. These attempt to comply with the criteria laid down in the Vatican's *Instruction on Respect for Human Life and its Origin and on the Dignity of Procreation (Donum vitae)*. The first procedure, called GIFT, is similar to IVF in that ovulating agents are used to produce multiple eggs. The eggs are retrieved by laparoscopy or by laparotomy and inserted along with washed semen into the fallopian tubes. Conception, therefore, occurs in the body (in vivo). It is also possible that donor eggs and/or sperm may be used with pregnancy established via GIFT in patients who had undergone premature ovarian failure. At least one open tube is required as well as ovaries accessible by laparoscopy or laparotomy.[22]

The second procedure, TOT, can be practised in two ways. In the first methodology there is ovarian stimulation with laporviconic oocyte retrieval just prior to ovulation, followed by only oocyte replacement into the lower portion of the fallopian tubes either hysteroscopically or by laparotomy. The married couple then have intercourse at home just prior to laparoscopy and also the day after. While the second is similar to, but more restrictive than GIFT, as no donor sperm are used and the sperm must be collected in a perforated elastic sheath during the conjugal act of intercourse, it also insists on the following procedures:

1   The conjugal act of intercourse using a perforated elastic sheath.
2   The separation of the husband's sperm from the wife's egg until the gametes are deposited into the fallopian tubes.
3   Conception occurs in the body, in vivo; since no embryos are formed, there is no chance of embryo manipulation, selection or discarding.

TOT, which was approved by the Pope John Center of the United States, appears to offer Catholic infertile couples, as well as Catholic medical institutions a viable alternative to the other reproductive techniques.[23]

Egg donation, embryo transfer and embryo freezing

Due to the complexity of infertility a number of reproduction-aiding procedures may be used in conjunction with IVF.[24] One of these is egg donation, which is simply the retrieval of eggs from one woman and their implantation into another. Egg donation might be practised on a woman whose ovaries are damaged but whose uterus is capable of normal functioning. Still, egg donation requires extensive hormonal regulation, for without the ability to freeze eggs or embryos readily, two women's cycles must be synchronised so that the donor ovulates at the time the recipient is ready to receive the egg. An attraction of this technology is that a woman, even though not the genetic agent of the child, can be both the gestational and the social parent.

Embryo transfer, in essence, is the transfer of a developing fertilised egg before implantation from one woman to another. The second woman gestates the embryo and ultimately gives birth. In the most common variant of this still rare technique, the first woman is artificially inseminated with sperm from the recipient's husband. The embryo is removed from the donor by the technique of lavage, that is, by flooding the uterus with a solution introduced and recovered through a catheter. It is then implanted into the gestational and social mother. It is, therefore, similar to egg donation.

It may also be used by women with normal ovaries but a dysfunctional uterus; husband and wife can initiate fertilisation naturally or by AIH, and the resulting embryo can be transferred to the uterus of a surrogate mother. Though embryo transfer is much easier than IVF in that it can be done in the physician's office without anaesthesia or surgery, the cycles of the two women still need to be synchronised and there is always the danger that lavage will lead to uterine infection.

Another emerging technique, embryo freezing, offers a number of technological advantages. The first successful human birth from a frozen embryo was in 1983. The baby was born to an Australian mother who had miscarried during an attempt at IVF but who successfully bore a child from an embryo frozen at her request as a precaution during the initial attempt. Development of the ability to freeze and then thaw embryos at a later date frees IVF and embryo transfer from certain time constraints: embryo transfer no longer requires synchronisation of two women's cycles, and a woman can store embryos for multiple attempts at implantation without further need to collect eggs, or as insurance against damage to her eggs or reproductive organs. Embryo freezing also offers the option of storing excess fertilised embryos rather than destroying them. From time to time the media reports the birth of a child which is the result of in vitro fertilisation and the freezing of the embryo. Therefore it is quite possible to have two or more children of identical conception age, but differing birth ages.

Need for donated eggs

At present there is a shortage of donated eggs, and women who need them often face a very long wait for treatment. In Britain and in other countries where IVF and experimentation is permitted, donated eggs can be used to create embryos for research if they are used to promote advances in the treatment of infertility, increased knowledge about the causes of congenital diseases and the causes of miscarriages, develop more effective techniques of contraception, and develop methods of detecting the presence of gene or chromosome abnormalities in embryos before implantation.[25]

Presently the current method of obtaining mature eggs involves adult women in intrusive and uncomfortable medical procedures which are not without risks. The donor needs to take drugs to stimulate the production of several mature eggs. Currently egg donors are women undergoing sterilisations or women who have surplus eggs after fertility treatment. Occasionally friends or relatives of a recipient will donate eggs, but usually women donate anonymously, simply inspired by the desire to help other women who are infertile.

To remedy this egg shortage it is proposed that ovarian tissue from adults, cadavers and aborted fetuses may be used. The use of donated adult, cadaveric or fetal ovarian tissue could provide many more eggs for IVF and embryo research than are currently available. There are thousands of immature eggs in fetal ovaries and large numbers in the normally fertile adult women which have the potential to ripen into mature eggs.

There are three major actual or potential uses of immature oocytes or ovarian tissue. They are:

Immature oocytes—in the future it may be possible to mature eggs obtained from donated ovarian tissue from patients and cadavers for use in treatment or research. A South Korean group has already reported that this can be done with ovarian tissue from patients. Live births have resulted in this Korean research.[26] However, it is not yet an established clinical practice. In addition, research done on animals has reached a stage which suggests that adult human ovarian tissue or that from cadavers could become a potential source of eggs in the future.

Ovarian tissue grafting—grafting of functional ovarian tissue has been carried out experimentally for nearly a hundred years.[27] Currently development of this technique in humans is directed towards helping women who are likely to become sterile as a result of cancer therapy, using their own tissue which may be removed before therapy and replaced afterwards, so avoiding problems of tissue rejection. This is the female equivalent of a man in a similar position storing his own sperm. In theory donated grafted tissue could help women who are unable to produce their own eggs. The purpose of the grafting would be to allow women to produce eggs in the normal way but the eggs would be genetically the donor's. The biggest problem to be overcome would be that of rejection of the donated tissue.

Fetal ovarian tissue—successful transfer of ovarian tissue from mouse fetuses into recipient mice was achieved about fifty years ago resulting in live offspring.[28] Ovarian tissue from human aborted fetuses has not yet been used in this way. It is not yet known whether the early female eggs from such material could develop into mature eggs or be capable of giving rise to a baby after fertilisation. Scientists believe that being able to grow and mature human eggs from fetal ovarian tissue is still some way off, as is grafting of human fetal ovarian tissue.[29]

In the first six months of 1994 the British Human Fertilisation and Embryology Authority produced a consultative document on these issues and asked for comments from interested parties. Due to this consultation the Authority ruled in July 1994 that the use of eggs from aborted fetuses to enable infertile women to become pregnant was wrong and banned the procedure. Only eggs or ovarian tissue from live donors, who had given their consent, could be used in treating infertility. It also said that it could envisage the use of eggs from dead women—such as road accident victims—for infertility treatment 'in principle', but it would not approve their use at present. However, it allowed research on eggs or fetal tissue irrespective of whether they were taken from live donors, corpses or fetuses.[30] Research could produce great benefits, the authority felt, helping to alleviate disease, improving fertility treatment and preventing the passing on of inheritable disorders.

This decision ended the prospect of children being born whose 'mothers' were aborted fetuses. The reason given was that there were worries about the safety of the method, which is years from being fully developed, the strength of public opposition and the possible effects on children when learning of their origins.[31] This might have caused disappointment to some women who were willing to try this procedure. However, the scientific community got what it required as it ensured that experimentation could now continue using material which was previously unavailable.

Sex pre-selection

The reproduction-aiding technologies described so far aim at the birth of a child. Many other startling and far-reaching techniques are being developed for goals that are ancillary to the production of a child. One such goal is the prediction and selection of the traits of one's child. Particular energy is being spent in attempting to pre-select the child's sex.[32] Though claims have outstripped actual success, the ability to select one's child's sex has been growing.

Sex pre-selection is in fact quite an old endeavour, and a great deal of folklore tells how to ensure the birth of a boy or (less frequently) a girl. For example it has been held that the birth of a girl would be more likely if the mother ate sweet foods and a boy more likely if she ate sour foods, or alternatively, if boots were worn to bed or if the male hung his pants on the right side of the bed.

Most recent scientific attempts at sex pre-selection have sought to determine the child's sex by selecting for or giving advantage to the type of sperm that would fertilise the egg (sperm carrying an X chromosome for females, and a Y chromosome for males). While controversy exists, several differences between sperm carrying X chromosomes and those carrying Y chromosomes have been proposed: the former are larger, more dense, slower moving, and inhibited by alkaline environments, whereas the latter die sooner, are more numerous in each ejaculation, and are slowed by acidic environments.

Although various techniques are proposed to differentiate the X and Y chromosomes, so far none has achieved widely acceptable success, but it is almost certain that the option of sex pre-selection is close at hand.[33]

As can be seen from this brief survey of reproduction-aided techniques many moral questions arise. Apart from the techniques themselves and the possible use or disposal of spare embryos there are more fundamental questions which need to be addressed. Does the use of aided-reproduction dehumanise the people directly involved in the wonder of procreation? What effect does it have on the relationship of a couple who resort to one of these procedures, especially if a donor is employed as in the case of artificial insemination and surrogacy? Are these procedures just another mechanism for re-enforcing a patriarchal domination of women? Are women in danger of being viewed as just vessels for reproduction which is determined primarily by men? What is the potential effect on the children who are conceived in this way? Is there not a danger that children will be looked at as just another commodity which can be tailored to our required needs? All these are complex questions for which there are no easy answers. But if society wishes to proceed with aided-reproduction it needs to confront them openly and honestly.

WHY EXPERIMENT ON EMBRYOS?

There is no doubt that scientific discoveries require experimentation: this holds true within medical science as in all scientific fields. A brief survey of the research and experimentation necessary to achieve an in vitro conception, implantation and maturity to birth supports this claim. However, what is now being proposed, within medical science, is a new range of experiments on the early human embryo. What are the hoped-for benefits of these new experiments?

On one level these experiments could be seen as facilitating the acquiring of new and important knowledge about the process of fertilisation and perfecting the in vitro procedure. It could also assist in solving questions concerning male and female infertility. It is possible that new methods to prevent fertilisation, i.e. contraception, could also be developed. On another level it is hoped that a better understanding of the causes of birth defects in children will be uncovered. If we are able to understand the causes of these defects, we might also be able to remedy them.

However, critics of laboratory research with early embryos argue that such research is not compatible with the kind of respect that should be shown to developing embryos who have the potential to become human beings. Contrary viewpoints on the ethics of human embryo research are clearly based on differing conceptions of the moral status of the early human embryo. The public policy debate on this question has raged in several countries with no clear resolution. Most public bodies charged with reaching a judgment on human embryo research have found the research to be ethically acceptable, in principle, if it is intended to develop important knowledge that cannot be gained in any other way.[34]

Over the past number of years various types of experimental aspirations and procedures have been brought into the public domain by the media. Some of these reports have been factual, while others have been purely fictional. The following section proposes to examine what experiments are currently being engaged in, what possible future developments could emerge, and to dispel some of the fictional scenarios that are currently reported by certain sections of the media.

New directions in experimentation

Advances in the pre-natal diagnosis of many genetic disorders have accelerated in the past few years. In the early days chromosomal analysis and certain biochemical tests were the mainstay of pre-natal diagnosis. All this has now changed with the advent of numerous genetic probes to detect the presence or absence of a large number of normal or mutated genes within the genome. This technology means that a single cell biopsy of early human embryos grown by in vitro fertilisation is now possible. The DNA[35] can be identified and screened using a panel of DNA probes in order to detect the presence or absence of a variety of normal or mutated genes. This opens up two further possibilities. First, a panel of embryos generated by in vitro fertilisation could be screened and the 'best' one returned to the mother for re-implantation and further development. Second, specific gene therapy to correct various genetic defects is achievable as embryos carrying such defects can now be detected.[36] These procedures could allow embryos to be screened not only for major genetic diseases but also for a variety of other characteristics including such things as susceptibility to adult cancers, infection, sex and height. Scientists could then attempt to perform some type of corrective medication of these genetic defects. In 1982 Dr French Anderson introduced the four well-known categories of human gene therapy into scientific literature. This type of correction falls into four basic categories:

1 Somatic cell gene therapy;
2 Germ-line therapy;
3 Enhancement genetic engineering; and
4 Eugenic genetic engineering.

Somatic cell gene therapy

This type of genetic intervention would aim to cure a condition that is generally acknowledged to be a disease by genetically altering the non-reproductive cells of a patient. In such cases of somatic gene therapy, the effect of the transplant stays with the individual and cannot be passed on to their children. Thus, for example, if a particular gene were detected in an individual embryo this gene could be re-inserted into the correct stem cell line thus correcting the genetic defect and preventing a major adult handicap.[37] The first successful case of human gene therapy was in 1990, when Michael Blaese and his colleagues at the US National Institute of Health transplanted a correct gene into a girl whose immune system lacked a vital protein—adenosine deaminase (ADA).[38] ADA deficiency is one of a category of inherited disorders in which a person's immune system is found to be incapable of challenging infections. Its most famous victim was David, who was portrayed by the actor John Travolta in the television film *The Boy in the Plastic Bubble*. David eventually died.

There are a number of possibilities with somatic line gene therapy. For example, a patient's bone marrow cells could have a defect corrected in the laboratory and then put back into their body to provide the missing enzyme. Or a cancer patient could have tumour cells removed to be modified with genes for growth factors in such a way that when re-inoculated, they stimulate the patient's immune system to destroy the cancer. If disorders of this type could be corrected by gene therapy not only would the life-span of the patient be enhanced, but also their quality of life.

These techniques are sophisticated and technically demanding, but they do not differ in principle from other forms of disease treatment. They do not in any way affect a person's inheritance, and raise no significant new moral questions. This point was stressed in an editorial in *The Lancet* in January 1989.

Why does gene therapy seem to raise major ethical issues when only somatic cells are involved? It cannot be because new genetic material is being introduced into the patient since organ and bone marrow transplants do just that routinely. Moreover, treatments with radiation and certain drugs will cause alterations in the genetic material. Neither can it be the safety argument since there is no reason to believe that gene therapy will be more dangerous than a host of other treatments. All new medical interventions carry risks and there are well established procedures for introducing, for example, new drugs. It is hard to see how anyone could object to curing disabling genetic diseases.[39]

Indeed, it would be unethical not to implement gene therapy for patients with life-threatening ailments, argues Dr French Anderson, one of its pioneers. 'Patients with serious genetic disease have little other hope at present for alleviation of their medical problems. Arguments that genetic engineering might some day be misused do not justify the needless perpetuation of human suffering caused by unnecessarily delaying this potentially powerful therapeutic procedure.'[40]

Used simply to cure disease, somatic gene therapy raises relatively few problems from a moral and public policy point of view: anyone who accepts organ transplantation should find little moral difference between that and the transplantation of a gene. Moral problems arise when gene therapy is applied not to the treatment of a recognisable disease, but to the enhancement of existing traits; not to rectify nature's mistakes, but to improve upon nature.[41]

Germ-line manipulation
Unlike somatic line manipulations germ-line manipulations are likely to be almost exclusively at the DNA level. Here a genetic defect in the germ, or reproductive cells of a patient, are corrected so that the offspring of the patient inherits the correction. In recent years the technology for such manipulation has advanced dramatically in experimental animals. Within animal experimentation a transgenetic animal or plant is one whose genetic composition has been altered to include selected DNA sequences from other organisms by methods other than those used in conventional animal breeding. The most usual method for introducing the non-parented DNA is by injecting into one of the pronuclei of the early embryo. Such techniques are relatively straightforward in mice but more difficult in domestic species such as sheep, cattle, pigs and probably in humans. These transgenetic techniques have enabled scientists to develop new strains of organisms of benefit to the agricultural and medical industries. These include the production of organisms genetically resistant to disease, the development of more efficient domesticated livestock, e.g. to get animals to grow faster, bigger and at a high food conversion ratio without upsetting the physiological balance. Another result would be the production of animals capable of existing in an adverse environment, e.g. by engineering in genes which confer resistance to certain environmental hazards such as heavy metals.[42]

However, this type of therapy in humans would be extremely difficult as it would require that we learn how to insert a gene not only into the appropriate cells of the patient's body, but also how to introduce it into the germ-line of the patient in such a way that it would be transmitted to offspring and would be functional in the correct way in the correct cells of the offspring. At present, modifying the germ-line might seem ridiculously unlikely. But the rapid progress in somatic line gene therapy demonstrates that it would be unwise to underestimate the rapid progress of science. The question is, should it be applied to the human embryo?

Enhancement genetic engineering

This is no longer therapy of a genetic disorder, it is the insertion of an additional normal gene (or a gene modified in a specific way) to produce a change in some characteristic that the individual wants. Enhancement would involve the insertion of a single gene, or a small number of genes, that would produce the desired effect; for example, greater size through the insertion of an additional growth hormone gene into the cells of an embryo.[43] Professor Ferguson suggests that it might be possible to insert different gene codings for antibodies against all major infections, including hepatitis B, malaria, AIDS etc.[44] Currently single gene replacement therapy is feasible; multiple gene replacement and other developments can only be predicted for the future.

Eugenic genetic engineering

This has received considerable attention in the popular press, with the result that at times unjustified fears have been produced because of claims that scientists might soon be able to re-make human beings. In fact, however, such traits as personality, character, formation of body organs, fertility, intelligence, physical, mental and emotional characteristics etc. are enormously complex. Dozens, perhaps hundreds, of unknown genes that interact in totally unknown ways probably contribute to each such trait. The effect of environmental influences on genetic backgrounds is at present poorly understood. With time, as more is learned about each of these complex traits, individual genes that play specific roles will be discovered. Undoubtedly disorders will be recognised that are caused by defections in these genes. Then, somatic cell gene therapy could be employed to correct the defect. But the concept of 're-making a human' (i.e. eugenic genetic engineering) is not realistic at present.[45]

Germ-line enhancement and eugenic therapy can be viewed in both a positive and negative light. It can be argued that the removal of a fatal gene from the human gene pool would be beneficial to humanity. A good example of this would be the removal of the Huntington's chorea gene from the biological legacy of a family. Gene therapy of this type is commonly called negative germ-line therapy, because it involves the removal of unwanted or dangerous genes. This type of germ-line therapy does not particularly worry observers. But it is the positive version of germ-line therapy, the addition of attributes, that causes the most concern. At issue is the extent to which we could use this technology to improve intelligence or modify inherited make-ups in desirable but unpredictable ways. Could we eventually arrive at the point of genetic supermarkets where parents could select the characteristics of their forthcoming child?

Even when discussing enhancement germ-line therapy it is necessary to differentiate between what would be considered appropriate and what would not. Perhaps the addition of height genes to small people, or for hair to the bald, or good eyesight to the myopic might be considered appropriate, while genes to enhance intelligence or athleticism might be inappropriate. The reason for this would be that it would violate the notion of the sanctity of human individuality which seems to be at the core of the individuality of persons. How we begin to differentiate between what we consider negative and positive therapy is a matter for research and common discussion. The United States Institute of Medicine and National Academy of Sciences makes this clear in its report on human gene therapy.

The prospect of parents turning to enhancement techniques to produce perfect children raises important questions about the value of the individual in our society and about the appropriate use of limited health care resources.[46]

What, therefore, is needed is a calm appraisal of genetic engineering. The term 'genetic engineering' is convenient, but unfortunately it is also emotive and confusing. In the public's mind, it muddles all the different applications of DNA technology. It is a point emphasised by the *Lancet* editorial which makes the point that 'it is curious how frightened people are of genetic engineering compared with, say child abuse'. It goes on to point out that genetic engineering has so far damaged no one. By contrast, smoking, AIDS, drug and alcohol abuse have caused massive damage to children in utero. What is needed is an educated public. They need to be sufficiently DNA-literate before they make decisions which could affect the many benefits of germ-line manipulation.[47]

In referring back to Dr French Anderson's basic categories it is enhancement and eugenic genetic engineering which therefore cause the most concern. The core of this concern is 'the slippery slope leading to attempts at germ-line enhancement that causes all of us to question whether a strict prohibition at the germ-line might not be the safest course . . .'[48] Nevertheless, French Anderson remains a strong supporter of germ-line gene therapy, at least as long as we are able to distinguish therapy from enhancement. The line between ethical and unethical genetic interventions is, according to French Anderson, clearly to be sought in the distinction between what is therapy and what is not therapy. Moreover, since 1983, he seems to consistently suggest that only therapy of the most severe genetic diseases be allowed.[49]

Embryonic/fetal transplantations
The use of embryonic or fetal cells or tissues to transplant into other embryos or fetuses or adults is a current reality. The first point to make on this issue is that such fetal therapy can be conducted regardless of in vitro fertilisation techniques. In many instances cells or tissues have come from embryos or fetuses

which are much older than the age to which human embryos are currently being developed in vitro. Theoretically it is possible that embryos derived from in vitro fertilisation procedures could be grown up to the maximum stage and then the required cells or tissues removed and further grown in cells or organ culture until they were at the correct stage for transplantation. Pragmatically, however, it is much easier to remove such cells or tissues from embryos undergoing elective or therapeutic abortion. Two major types of transplant situations can be envisaged.

The first is embryo to adult. In this situation embryonic cells or tissues could be introduced into the adult human in order to correct some failing system. In the simplest case, hormone secreting cells might be introduced to colonise a particular gland where the existing cells were either malfunctioning or had been destroyed. Such considerations would apply to diseases like diabetes and thyroid deficiency. In other circumstances grafts of tissue may be placed so as to restore some kind of function in particular areas. Both these types of manipulation have been conducted in experimental animals and in some cases already in humans. Moreover, in experimental animals whole organ transplants have been conducted from late fetuses into adults. Thus, transplantation of the fetal liver or the fetal heart or kidney may be conducted so as to augment the function of a failing adult organ. In these cases the transplant is not replacive, as in the conventional adult to adult transplant, but rather is additional to the failing adult organ, i.e. a supplementary transplant. Experiments in animals have shown that such transplants are highly successful. As the adult organ fails, so the fetal organ develops and begins to take over the function; moreover the surgery is nowhere near as traumatic as replacive transplants. It appears that increasing use will be made of fetal cells or tissues to replace or augment failing and diseased adult tissues. Such considerations have brought their own set of ethical problems, such as the diagnosis of death in an embryo, and the ethics of keeping alive human embryos which are incompatible with life after birth (e.g. anencephaly) so that valuable tissues might develop and be removed for adult transplantation.

The second category concerns embryo/fetus to embryo/fetus. The increasing sophistication of pre-natal ultrasonic diagnosis now means that it is possible to detect embryos or fetuses with structural malfunctions very shortly after these malfunctions have occurred. This implies that direct fetal therapy is possible. Such fetal therapy may involve administration of compounds such as amniotic fluid replacement or fetal blood transfusions; fetal surgery—either simple repair or insertion of a prosthesis (e.g. repair of cleft lip and cleft palate or spina bifida; the insertion of a drain into the brain in cases of hydronephrosis); or transplantations of organs or cells into the embryo. All these procedures have been conducted in experimental animals and many have been conducted in humans. It is evident that in the absence of any kind of therapy such embryos would die. Therefore, some scientists argue that any kind of intervention to save the embryo can be justified.[50]

Fictional scenarios

With the advent of reproductive-aided technology numerous wild scientific theories have emerged in the popular press. These have ensured that at times the public is frightened into believing that if science is given a free hand certain diabolical humans will be born. It might therefore prove helpful to dispel some of these fictional scenarios.

Cloning is one of these areas. The possibility of indefinitely cloning individuals, or the scenario of the mad dictator who wishes to populate the world with identical copies of him/herself are pure fiction from the scientific standpoint.

It has also been suggested that in vitro fertilisation techniques could be used to cross human gametes with those from other species to create human-animal hybrids. This is currently technically impossible, and is likely to remain so. One fictional scenario put forward as a worry of in vitro fertilisation is that it would be possible to grow embryos all the way through gestation outside the womb—ectogenesis. At present this is not achievable in any animal and indeed the problems are so complex that the future holds little hope of complete ectogenesis.

Other scenarios paint the picture of complex brain transplants from either one embryo into another or embryos into adults or even adults into adults. The complex connections within the central nervous system and from the central nervous system to the peripheral nervous system make any kind of large-scale brain transplantation next to impossible. It is certainly true that very small segments of the brain may be transplanted, e.g. cells may be placed in a particular area to restore function which had been lost through disease or trauma or ageing. However, complex brain transplants to change any individual's personality or intelligence are pure fiction from a scientific standpoint.[51]

While it is not clear precisely which kinds of research will be most useful, nor what other promising possibilities will arise in the future, we do know that none of them is likely to be realised without embryo research. John Harris therefore argues that if embryos can be used to save the lives of adults and children and for therapeutic and diagnostic purposes, we would require strong moral arguments to justify cutting ourselves off from these benefits with the consequent loss of life and perpetuation of pain and misery.[52] As mentioned during the introduction to this section a decision to experiment on human embryos will depend on what moral status is given to the embryo. This particular issue has raised considerable debate, with many conflicting views and opinions. What is decided in this instance could very well affect the future directions medicine will take.

THE MORAL STATUS OF THE EARLY HUMAN EMBRYO

Broadly speaking there are three principal viewpoints on the moral status of the early human embryo.[53] The first viewpoint asserts that human embryos are entitled to protection as human beings from the time of fertilisation forward. According to this view, any research or other manipulation, such as freezing, that damages any embryo or interferes with its prospects for transfer to a uterus and subsequent development is ethically unacceptable. This perspective on embryonic status is based on two kinds of factual evidence. First, the embryonic genotype is established at the time of fertilisation. Secondly, given the proper environment, early embryos have the potential to become full-term fetuses, children and adults.

A second viewpoint denies that early human embryos have any moral status. According to this view, we who are adult human beings have no moral obligations to early human embryos. This opinion also appeals to scientific evidence, especially the fact that only about 30 to 40% of embryos produced through human sexual intercourse develop to maturity in utero and are delivered as live infants.[54] It also notes that the biological individuality of the early embryo is established only toward the end of the first 14 days of development; before that time one embryo can divide into twins or, more rarely, two embryos with different genotypes can combine into a single hybrid embryo. Finally, this position argues that an undifferentiated entity like the early embryo which has no organs, no limbs, and no sentience, cannot have moral status.

The third viewpoint acknowledges that although early embryos demand moral recognition, the obligations that accompany this recognition can be outweighed by other moral duties, for example, the duty to develop new and better methods of providing care for infertile couples.[55]

Fertilisation as the beginning of a human individual

The first viewpoint reasons that fertilisation is the time at which full moral status is acquired. This argument tends to rely on the features of the fertilisation process, or on some of its aspects in combination with an emphasis on the potentiality of the newly formed entity.

The genetic argument pinpoints fertilisation as the time at which moral status is acquired. It is then that entities that 'are genetically human beings'[56] are created. For this argument the crucial event during fertilisation is the formation of a human genotype. It is claimed that only at fertilisation, and not before, does a new genetic member of the species *homo sapiens* come about, and at no other point in development is there any 'significant'[57] genetic change. This claim is often coupled with the basic moral principle that it is wrong to destroy innocent

human beings which, if taken to include the zygote, leads to the
conclusion that it is wrong to destroy early human life from the
moment of fertilisation.[58]

Arguments of this type have led its proponents to reason that
'we know that a new human individual organism with the
internal potential to develop into an adult, given nurture, comes
into existence as a result of the process of fertilisation at
conception.'[59] Events post-fertilisation are, therefore, envisaged
as comprising a continuum of developmental changes so that it
is impossible to isolate any one stage at which to attribute the
attainment of moral status. In contrast to this continuity,
fertilisation is seen as a radical discontinuity or 'transformation'
in development. Therefore the union of the two gametes to form
the single zygote at fertilisation is the only distinct stage at
which it can be claimed that a human entity begins to exist.
Proponents of this claim then argue that the fundamental moral
claim against killing are applicable from fertilisation, as this
event marks the time when an individual human being begins to
exist.

Professor John Marshall, who served on the Warnock
Committee which enquired into the ethical questions raised by in
vitro fertilisation, embryo experimentation and surrogacy,
argues that because a unique entity has come into existence at
fertilisation which has the potential to become a person it is
wrong to destroy it. He, therefore, rules out experimental
procedures which don't recognise this potential and result in the
destruction of the embryo.[60]

Those authors who oppose the view that a human individual
comes into existence at fertilisation also begin with an
examination of the fertilisation process and its completion. In his
book *When Did I Begin?* the Australian Catholic theologian,
Norman Ford, argues that at this early stage of post-fertilisation
development it is important to distinguish between the concept
of genetic and ontological individuality. Biologists, he observes,
tend to speak of genetic individuality as being synonymous with
the beginning of the human person. But, due to the potential
existence of identical twins, Ford argues, the genetic and

ontological identity or individuality cannot be seen as identical. The genetic code in the zygote does not suffice to constitute or define a human individual in an ontological sense. Identical twins have the same genetic code, but they are distinct ontological individuals. Failure to appreciate this significant distinction, according to Ford, could lead to a mistake in determining the timing of establishing the beginning of a human person.[61]

As additional evidence for his case Ford points to the fact that the embryonic genome is not switched on or activated in the human before the 2-cell stage, and probably not before the 4-cell stage, even though the embryonic genetic programme is established at the completion of fertilisation. The genetic programme is necessary for the emergence of a new human individual, but unless it is switched on it cannot come into existence. Ford therefore concludes that unless the blueprint of the DNA in the zygote's genotype is activated, it is practically a 'dead letter' and could not be considered a true human individual even if it does produce genetically identical progeny up to the second or fourth cell stage before degenerating.[62]

As already noted some authors argue that due to the developmental capacity of the zygote it should be treated as a human individual. But this viewpoint can be seriously challenged due to the possibility of monozygotic twinning. The zygote has the natural capacity to become one or more human beings by virtue of its own inherent active potential, when it cleaves through the process of mitosis into the first two cells or blastomeres. Like the zygote these two daughter cells are totipotent—each one can develop into a complete living human individual. Whatever the cause of monozygotic twinning in the zygote at the two cell stage, the fact that it cleaves into two individual blastomeres that may develop separately as identical twins does not mean the zygote itself is not a true ontological individual. But once it divides into two separate twin daughter blastomeres, it apparently ceases to exist and loses its ontological individuality to give rise to two new genetically identical, but distinct living ontological individuals. The continuity of the same ontological individual ceases when the zygote forms twins. The zygote is not the same ontological individual as either one of the eventual twins that result from its development notwithstanding its genetic identity continuing throughout all its subsequent cleavages.[63] Therefore Ford concludes that it is not a human being that loses its ontological individuality but only a human zygote when monozygotic twinning occurs at this early stage.[64] From these observations it could be concluded that a human individual could not be present at the completion of fertilisation.[65]

In his book, *Wonderwoman and Superman*, Professor John Harris argues that there are two objections to the potentiality argument for the moral significance of the embryo. The first is the fact that although an entity can undergo changes that will make it significantly different this does not constitute a reason for treating it as if it had already undergone those changes. We are all potentially dead, but no one supposes that this fact constitutes a reason for treating us as if we were already dead. The second objection is that if we regard as morally significant anything which has potential to become a fully fledged human being, then the egg and the sperm taken together but as yet un-united have the same potential as the fertilised egg.[66] This argumentation ignores the distinction between the potential of a new genetic individual and the potential to become a new genetic individual.

Related to the issue of potentiality is the question of parthenogenesis. This refers to the birth of the young without prior sexual intercourse and without the consequent union of the genetic complement of the ovum with that of the male sperm (i.e. the virgin birth). It occurs regularly in some vertebrates, such as fish and one strain of turkey, but probably does not naturally or spontaneously occur in any mammal. It has been experimentally induced up to mid-term gestation in mice. Mouse eggs can be activated by manipulation techniques employing the use of alcohol and electric shock to produce embryos. A parthenogenetic mouse fetus would have to be regarded as an ontological individual and consequently a true mouse at the fetal stage of development so long as it was still alive. Up to that point it develops and grows anatomically the same as any normal mouse.[67] Scientific literature does not report any verification of naturally occurring parthenogenetic development occurring in humans. There is some evidence that a secondary oocyte may begin spontaneous parthenogenetic development at the early stage of cleavage, but fails to result in organic development and soon perishes or gives rise to an ovarian teratoma.[68] Some IVF researches report cases of light-cell human embryos with only one set of chromosomes (i.e. 23x). These would have to be classed as examples of parthenogenetic development of human eggs.[69]

If we assume that a diploid parthenogenetic human embryo develops normally from the beginning, as in the case of mice, and if completion of fertilisation is taken as the beginning of the human being, we would have to conclude that the normally cleaving and developing parthenogenetic human embryo would likewise be a human being until it died. By the same token, the reasons used to argue that the human being does not begin at fertilisation would equally apply to argue that the human being does not begin when the human egg is parthenogenetically activated, either spontaneously or artificially. In other words, the phenomenon of parthenogenesis in humans does not per se throw any light on the question of when the human individual or person begins. These experimental possibilities, according to Ford, certainly add to the existing doubts about the completion of fertilisation as the beginning of the human individual simply on the grounds of egg activation and the genetic uniqueness that is established at that stage of human development.[70]

Some authors, Karen Dawson[71] and Patricia Jacobs, argue that due to the high loss of human fertilisations[72] at this early stage the case dependent on potentiality is further undermined. Jacobs reports that there is evidence that pregnancy losses are high in humans prior to the time when pregnancy is clinically recognised.[73] Up to 50% of ovulated eggs and zygotes recovered after operations were found to be so grossly abnormal that it would be very unlikely that they would result in viable pregnancies. She also suggests that 30% of conceptions abort spontaneously before these pregnancies are clinically verified. The scientific literature is not unanimous on the incidence of natural wastage prior to, and during, implantation in humans, varying from 15% to as much as 50%.[74] But there is evidence to suggest that the vast majority of these losses are due to chromosomal defects caused during gametogenesis and fertilisation.

Even if we accept that there is a high loss rate of embryos either before or after implantation can we therefore conclude that these embryos are not human? Before making this decision we need to seriously consider infant mortality. At times in human history infant morality was as high as 50%. Few people would doubt that these young children were not individual human persons.[75] Ford argues that one cannot reasonably conclude from this embryo loss rate that human embryos several weeks old could not be human on the grounds that this would conflict with the wisdom of Divine Providence.[76]

Human individuality after fertilisation

If it is accepted that a human individual does not start at fertilisation, when can it be assumed that this does take place? There are various compelling and equally convincing counter arguments that the human individual begins at implantation (13 days after fertilisation) or gastrulation[77] (from day 14 to about day 19 after fertilisation). Ford promotes the theory that it is the emergence of the primitive streak which determines the beginning of individual human life. He argues that 'after gastrulation, by the end of the third week when the neural folds have been formed and the primitive cardiovascular system is functioning to enable nutrition and growth as a whole to take place, there are sufficient reasons to justify asserting that a living individual with a human nature has been formed. Consequently, a human being or a person is present.'[78] As gastrulation develops at about day 14–15 a convergence of epiblastic cells occurs in the posterior part of the embryonic dice: this is called the primitive streak. It is a key factor, a primary organiser for the process of differentiation during gastrulation. Usually the cells piling up on the embryonic plate form only one primitive streak. Sometimes none is formed, with the result that no embryo develops. By the 16 day stage after fertilisation, all the cells derived from the zygotes have been committed to being part of extraembryonic structures or part of the embryo proper.[79] The appearance of one primitive streak signals that only one embryo proper has been formed and begun to exist. According to Ford, prior to this stage it would be pointless to speak about the presence of a true human being in an ontological sense. A human individual could scarcely exist before a definitive human body is formed.[80]

Keith Moore succinctly expresses the significance of the primitive streak in embryological terms. He writes, 'when the primitive streak appears, it is possible to identify the embryo's craniocaudal axis, its cranial and caudal ends, its dorsal and ventral surfaces, and its right and left sides.'[81]

Anne McLaren comes to a similar conclusion. She begins by stating that

if we are talking not about the origin of life . . . but about the origin of an individual life, one can trace back directly from the newborn baby to the foetus, and back further to the origin of the individual embryo at the primitive streak stage in the embryonic plate at sixteen or seventeen days. If one tries to trace back further than that there is no longer a coherent entity. Instead there is a larger collection of cells, some of which are going to take part in the subsequent development of the embryo and some of which aren't.[82]

Therefore, the sort of individuation and multicellular unity displayed with the appearance of the primitive streak justifies the claim that this is the beginning of an individual being that is a human person with the potential to develop to the age of reason.[83]

Ford goes on to propose that at this stage of the formation of the primitive streak the human individual would be ensouled with a rational soul or life-principle since it has the form of the human body, i.e. it makes the human body be the same individual from that stage until death.[84] Support for this thinking is found in Professors Berry and Mahoney. Professor Berry, an evangelical geneticist, argues that 'it is a false extrapolation to assume that "life" from God which transforms a biological being into a spiritual one is automatically given to every fertilised egg'.[85] The Catholic theologian Professor John Mahoney writes that

> only the conclusions to be drawn from the facts of actual or possible twinning and combination of fertilised eggs appear to resist critical examination and to indicate that, rather than ensoulment occurring at the stage of conception, it can take place only when there is an unambiguously individual subject capable of receiving the soul by virtue of the fact that it is passing beyond the stages of simple reduplication and is beginning to ramify and diversify through the development of its bodily organs.[86]

Dr Teresa Iglesias believes that the conclusions arrived at thus far are a distortion of the true scientific picture. Due to the imprecision of our empirical knowledge of monozygotic twinning and the mechanisms of embryonic 'fusing' or recombination, conclusions which affect personal and public morality should not so easily be drawn. She goes on to argue in favour of viewing the embryo as a living whole, which neither divides nor fuses with another whole being, as a whole being, although some of its parts (cells) can do so. This means that there can be fragmentation of living beings giving rise to asexual generation. If there is no 'fusion' or 'splitting' of living beings as total wholes then the question of a non-coherent entity or organically 'unstable' embryos does not arise. Therefore, according to Iglesias, stable individuality remains a feature of every living being considered as a whole even though it can shed cells which can become part of other organisms through grafting and transplantation. It can also shed cells to become a new living being, either on its own or in combination with another cell or cells. Although the living being can be deprived of or damaged in substantial organic parts, yet it will internally regulate the deficiency and continue to live and develop as well as a well-functioning whole through the powers of regulation, regeneration and healing. It follows that if the early embryo, as a living whole, is an individual stable organism it appears that the possibility of twinning and recombination in every conceptus does not argue against a biologically stable subject for immediate animation or ensoulment.[87]

It is evident from the extensive literature on the subject of the moral status of the early embryo that convincing arguments exist for attributing full moral status at the moment of fertilisation and for stating that the primitive streak is the beginning of an individual being that is a human person with the potential to develop to the age of reason. Due to these opposing views moral theology could be inclined to take a cautious approach and argue for full moral status at the moment of fertilisation, thus ruling out any form of manipulation. However, this would be to ignore the very real needs of infertile couples. Rather it could be argued that although early embryos demand moral recognition, the obligations that accompany this recognition can be outweighed by the moral duty to develop new and better methods of providing care for infertile couples. This would ensure that moral theology took an active part in assessing the morality of certain in vitro and experimental procedures.

HOW SOME WOMEN HAVE REACTED TO THE NEW TECHNIQUES OF AIDED REPRODUCTION

Considering that the major percentage of people affected by the new techniques of reproduction are women, it would be unjust if we did not mention some of their reactions to these new developments. It has been argued that women's biological and existing social arrangement have burdened women with bearing and rearing children, thereby robbing them of opportunities to become fully aware of and able to exercise their capabilities as human beings. Technological developments, such as contraception and abortion, which increased women's control over the reproductive process, were welcomed by most in the women's movements, and at first, innovations in reproductive technology were hailed as having the potential to free women from the 'tyranny of their biology'. However, a critical problem for the women's movement, especially in regard to social policy, is reconciling the feminist position that individual women should have freedom of choice in reproductive matters with the recognition that these choices can be informed by and re-enforce values that are antithetical to women's fulfilment. Many in the women's movement see the new techniques of aided reproduction as another means of male domination and manipulation. But it can also be argued that it is not the techniques themselves that are damaging to women, but rather the consciousness with which they are regarded. If this is the case then feminist critics should not oppose the techniques themselves, but instead should aim to change our culture and individual consciousness so that we are properly receptive to them.

Surrogate motherhood

Surrogate motherhood presents an enormous challenge for feminists. For some feminists, the argument against surrogacy is a simple one: it demeans us all as a society to sell babies. Surrogate motherhood has been described by its opponents not only as the buying and selling of children but as reproductive prostitution, reproductive slavery, the renting of a womb, incubating servitude, etc. The women who are surrogates are labelled paid breeders, biological entrepreneurs, breeder women, reproductive meat, interchangeable parts in the birth machinery, human incubates and prostitutes. Their husbands are seen, alternatively, as pimps or cuckolds. The children conceived according to a surrogacy agreement have been called chattels or merchandise to be expected in perfect condition.[88]

   The second line of argument opposes surrogacy because of the potential psychological and physical risks that it presents for women. It is considered unnatural for a mother to give up her child. This conclusion is arrived at because it has been found that, as birth mothers in traditional adoption situations often regret relinquishing their children, surrogate mothers must therefore feel the same way. But surrogate mothers are making their decisions about relinquishment under much different circumstances. The biological mother in the traditional situation is already pregnant as part of a personal relationship of her own. In many instances she would like to keep the child, but cannot because the relationship is not supportive or she cannot afford to raise the child herself. She generally feels that the relinquishment was forced upon her by either her parents, a counsellor or her lover.[89] The biological mother in the surrogate situation seeks out the opportunity to carry a child that would not exist were it not for the couple's desire to create a child as part of their relationship. She makes her decision in advance of pregnancy for internal, not externally enforced reasons. While 75% of the biological mothers who give a child up for adoption later change their minds, only around 1% of the surrogates have similar changes of heart.[90]

Some surrogate mothers argue that they are able to make these difficult choices. One of them claims: 'I find it extremely insulting that there are people saying that, as a woman I cannot make an informed choice about a pregnancy that I carry'; she continues by pointing out that she, like everyone else, 'makes other difficult choices in her life.'[91]

The third line of argument opposes surrogacy because of the potential harm it represents to potential children. One line of argument against surrogacy is that it is like adoption, and adoption harms children. However, such an argument is not sufficiently borne out in fact. There is evidence that adopted children do as well as non-adopted children in terms of adjustment and achievement. A family of two biological parents does not necessarily assure a child's well-being.

Another argument about potential harm to the resulting children is that parents will expect more of a surrogate child because of the £6,500 they have spent on his/her creation. But many couples spend more than that on infertility treatments without evidence that they expect more of the child. A caesarian section costs twice as much as natural childbirth, yet the parents don't expect twice as much of the children.[92]

Admittedly there is the potential danger that surrogate mothers could be viewed only as reproductive vessels and exploited. But Lori Andrews argues that if we insist on legislation to either outlaw surrogacy or to severely restrict it, this legislation could rebound on the feminist movement. It could ensure a reversal of many of the achievements of feminism and retard the larger feminist agenda.[93]

Reproductive continuity

Gena Corea, a well-known feminist writer on this topic, argues that reproductive technologies are transforming the experience of motherhood and placing it under the control of men.[94] She deals extensively with the real meaning of a woman's 'consent' to in vitro fertilisation in a society in which men as a social group control not just the choices open to women, but also women's motivation to choose.[95]

She points out that although advocates of the technologies highlight that women now have new 'options' and 'choices', this is to assume a society in which there are no serious differences of power and authority between individuals. Where power differences do prevail, coercion (subtle or otherwise) is apt to prevail. She says that in the discussion of in vitro fertilisation the harm women have been subjected to through the Pill, IUDs, estrogen replacement therapy, tranquillisers, unnecessary hysterectomies and caesarean sections seems to be forgotten as if the old reproductive technologies and new ones arose out of two separate medical systems, one of which has a clear record of hurting women, another of which will help women. But in fact there is one system and one low valuation of women in it.[96]

She is extremely sceptical of the male agenda, pointing out that although today the language men employ in speaking of the use of reproductive technology on women differs from that employed in speaking of its use on animals, it may not always be so. Women may find that the connection men have made for centuries between women and animals still lives on in patriarchal minds just as it lives on in men's laws and practices. Women and animals remain part of nature to be conquered and subjugated.[97] Ultimately, according to Corea, the issue is not fertility, but the exploitation of women.[98]

Sex pre-selection

Tabitha Powledge presents the argument for the claim that sex pre-selection is 'the original sexist sin', because it makes 'the most basic judgment about the worth of a human being rest first and foremost on its sex'.[99] However, it is false to believe that all persons who would like to preselect the sex of their children believe that members of one sex are inherently more valuable. Some people, for instance, would like to have a son because they already have one or more daughters (or vice versa), and they would like to have at least one child of each sex. Others may believe that, because of their own personal background or circumstances they would be better parents to a child of one sex rather than the other. On the surface, at least, such persons need not be motivated by invidious sexist beliefs.[100]

It may, however, be argued that the desire to pre-select sex is always based on covert sexist beliefs. Michael Bayles notes that the desire for a child of a particular sex is often instrumental to the fulfilment of other desires, such as the desire that the family name be carried on. Such instrumental reasons for sex pre-selection, he argues, are always ultimately based upon irrational and sexist beliefs.[101] But are these reasons that irrational?

A pragmatic reason for sex-preference in northern India (and many other parts of the world) is that a son is an economic asset, whereas a daughter usually is not. Because of sex discrimination in the job market, a daughter will almost certainly earn far less than a son. If the family is well-to-do, she is apt not to enter the job market at all. Thus, she will not be able to contribute much to her family's economic support; furthermore, the cost of providing her with a dowry is likely to be extremely high. Without a large dowry she will probably be unable to marry, and will remain dependent upon her family. If she does marry without a dowry that is considered suitably large, she may be tormented or murdered by her husband or in-laws. Under these conditions it would be difficult to show that the desire to have sons rather than daughters is irrational. In a similar way it would certainly be wrong to condemn the decision of a couple not to have children because they judge that they cannot afford to raise them. Why, then, should we condemn their decision not to have daughters for the same reason?[102]

Numerous speculations have been made about the long-term consequences should an effective means of sex pre-selection become widely available. Some authors have welcomed sex pre-selection as a voluntary means of reducing the birth rate and the number of unwanted children born in the attempt to get one of the 'right' sex, while others argue that the results are likely to be primarily detrimental. They fear that females may be psychologically harmed by the implementation of sex-preferences. There have been hundreds of studies purporting to prove or disprove the effects between birth order and such personality traits as initiative, creativity, anxiety, dependence, conservatism, rebelliousness, authoritarianism, mental illness, criminality and alcoholism. However, among the most consistent findings are that firstborns do achieve more in terms of formal education and career, but tend to be more dependent and affiliative.[103] Cecile Ernst and Jules Angst, Swiss psychologists, believe that there are some differences in the socialisation process undergone by firstborns and late-borns. But they conclude that these differences 'do not seem to leave indelible traces that can be predicted.'[104]

Equally disturbing are the possible social consequences of the sex ratio increases, i.e. increases in the relative number of males. An undersupply of women might result in their being increasingly confined to subordinate 'female' roles and/or subjected to increased male violence. Due to these fears Dharma Kumar reasons that a society with a balanced sex ratio is happier than one with a large preponderance of one sex or another. However, since most people, particularly in India and China, prefer boys to girls, if they are allowed to choose the sex of their child, an unbalanced sex ratio will result, so people must not be allowed to choose. He claims that a loss in individual freedom of choice (and short-term happiness) of a few is outweighed by the unhappiness of an unbalanced society.[105]

There is, according to Powledge, a predictable benefit of sex pre-selection that does much to counter-balance its possible ill effects. Fewer children will be doomed to abuse and neglect because they are of the 'wrong' sex—in most cases, because they are female. We will never know, she writes, how many short and miserable lives will be avoided through sex pre-selection, but the data on different mortality rates for female children in northern India and many other parts of the world suggest that the number would be quite significant.[106]

THE ATTITUDE OF THE CHRISTIAN COMMUNITY TO THE NEW AIDED REPRODUCTIVE TECHNOLOGIES

In vitro fertilisation and the accompanying experimentation on human embryos has raised important moral difficulties for the Christian community. The various Christian churches, due to their different theological approaches, have dealt with these questions in a variety of ways. An exploration of these different approaches may assist individuals to make better informed decisions when judging the morality of either IVF or embryo experimentation.

The Roman Catholic Church

One of the first responses to the issue of in vitro fertilisation was given by the Catholic Bishops' Joint Committee on Bio-Ethical Issues on behalf of the Roman Catholic Bishops of Great Britain to the Warnock Committee. In this document entitled, *In Vitro Fertilisation: Morality and Public Policy* they stated that 'they see no reason to consider "the simple case" of IVF as morally unacceptable'.[107] What they meant by 'the simple case', was the case in which sperm and egg are obtained from the husband and wife respectively and not from a third party (or donor) and no intentional destruction of the embryos is involved. However, due to the possibility of a misunderstanding that the bishops were actually approving of IVF in 'the simple case' a further clarification was issued. They went on to state that they 'did not give approval to the present practice of in vitro fertilisation within marriage. This they considered to be unacceptable because the process involves the intentional destruction of human embryos.' Yet they did not exclude the possibility that with further developments in the IVF technologies the factors which make it currently immoral could be remedied.[108]

The reason for the committee's opposition to in vitro fertilisation was due to what they considered to be the in-built significance of the IVF procedure, and the possible effects this would have on IVF parents, despite their high motivation. They argued that to choose to have a child by IVF was to choose to have a child as a product of human making. A relationship of this type would be one of radical inequality and profound subordination. Thus, the committee stated that the choice to have or to create a child by IVF is a choice in which the child does not have the status which the child of a 'normal' sexual union has. In this instance the status is of radical equality with the parents, and is a partnership with them in the familial community.[109]

The flaw they saw in the IVF process was that it separated procreation from sexual intercourse. If the child is to come into existence as an equal partner in the life of the couple these two aspects could not be separated.[110]

In March 1987 the Congregation for the Doctrine of the Faith responded to the developments of IVF with a much fuller explanation of the Catholic position in their document, *Instruction on Respect for Human Life in its Origin and on the Dignity of Procreation (Donum Vitae)*. The document taught that in vitro fertilisation is always morally wrong. The reasons for this position are based on the following premises:

1   there is an inseparable connection, willed by God and unable to be broken by persons on their own initiative, between the life-giving and love-giving meanings of the conjugal act;

2   to conceive or desire a child as a product of a technique and not as the fruit of the conjugal act is to treat the child as if he/she were an object or product; and

3   the 'language of the body' requires that the child be given
     life only in the personal bodily and spiritual act whereby
     husband and wife become 'one flesh' and express in a
     unique and proper way their personal and exclusive love for
     one another.[111]

When discussing the inseparability of the procreative and
unitive meanings of the marital act *Donum Vitae* begins by citing
Humanae Vitae which affirms

> the 'inseparable connection, willed by God and unable to be
> broken by man of his own initiative, between the two
> meanings of the conjugal act: the unitive meaning and the
> procreational meaning. Indeed, by its intimate structure, the
> conjugal act, while most closely uniting husband and wife,
> makes them capable of the generation of new lives, according
> to laws inscribed in the very being of man and woman'.[112]

Hence 'the conjugal act specific to the love between spouses' is
at once proper to nature and morally normative.[113] Similarly, it is
argued that surrogate motherhood is 'morally wrong because it
violates the biological and spiritual unity of husband and wife
and the parental relationship of parents and child.'[114]

Two categories of IVF are distinguished. One category is
homologous artificial fertilisation, which separately procures
eggs and sperm from a married couple, which are used to
produce a fertilised egg in vitro with subsequent embryo transfer
(ET) to the biological mother. The second category is
heterologous artificial fertilisation which separately procures
either donor eggs and/or donor sperm with subsequent embryo
transfer, either to the egg donor (the biological mother) or to a
surrogate womb (a non-biological source of the eggs). The
official teaching is that both forms of IVF are immoral because
both violate the dignity of the natural procreative act between
husband and wife.[115] It arrives at this conclusion by affirming,
with Pope Pius XII, that 'it is never permitted to separate these
different aspects to such a degree as positively to exclude either
the procreative intention [as is done in contraceptive intercourse]

or the conjugal relation'.[116] *Donum Vitae* then draws the following conclusion that 'fertilisation is licitly sought when it is the result of a "conjugal act which is per se suitable for the generation of children to which marriage is ordered by its nature and by which the spouses become one flesh". But from the moral point of view procreation is deprived of its proper perfection when it is not desired as the fruit of the conjugal act, that is to say, of the specific act of the spouses' union.'[117]

In short, *Donum Vitae* teaches that deliberately to separate the unitive and procreative meanings of the conjugal act is always wrong. Since homologous in vitro fertilisation requires such a deliberate separation of these meanings, it follows that this mode of generating human life is always morally wrong. This position is not the private property of Roman Catholicism. The influential Protestant writer Paul Ramsey was in full agreement with this position. In his book *Fabricated Man*[118] he equated IVF with genetic manipulation and argued against it.[119]

The second line of reasoning set forth in *Donum Vitae* supports the thesis that in vitro fertilisation violates the dignity of the child conceived. It argues that the child 'cannot be desired or conceived as the product of an intervention of medical or biological techniques'. The reason being is that it would be equivalent to reducing him or her to an object of scientific technology. No one may subject the coming of a child into the world to conditions of technical efficacy which are to be evaluated according to standards of control and dominion.[120] *Donum Vitae* then concludes that

conception by in vitro fertilisation is the result of the technical action which presides over fertilisation. Such fertilisation is neither in effect achieved nor positively willed as the expression and fruit of a specific act of the conjugal union. In homologous IVF and ET, therefore, even if it is considered in the context of de facto existing sexual relations, the generation of the human person is objectively deprived of its proper perfection, namely, that of being the result and fruit of a conjugal act in which the spouses can become 'co-operators with God for giving life to a new person.'[121]

This argument can be summed up by saying that if one desires or causes a child to come into existence as a product of a technique, one is making the child an object or 'product'. But this is incompatible with the equality in personal dignity between the child and those who give it life. Yet this is precisely what in vitro fertilisation does. Therefore, such fertilisation is a morally inappropriate way of generating new human life.

A third reason given by *Donum Vitae* to support the conclusion that in vitro fertilisation is morally wrong is based on its understanding of the 'language of the body'. Here the document first observes that

> spouses mutually express their personal love in the 'language of the body', which clearly involves both 'spousal meanings' and parental ones. The conjugal act by which the couple mutually express their self-gift at the same time expresses openness to the gift of life. It is an act that is inseparably corporal and spiritual. It is in their bodies and through their bodies that the spouses consummate their marriage and are able to become father and mother.

It then continues by saying that,

> in order to respect the language of their bodies and their natural generosity, the conjugal union must take place with respect for its openness to procreation; and the procreation of a person must be the fruit and result of married love. The origin of the human being thus follows from a procreation that is 'linked to the union, not only biological but also spiritual, of the parents, made one by the bond of marriage'. Fertilisation achieved outside of the bodies of the couple remains by this very fact deprived of the meanings and values which are expressed in the language of the body and the union of human persons.[122]

According to this argument in vitro fertilisation, which occurs outside the bodies of husband and wife and outside the bodily act in which their marital union is uniquely and properly expressed, is a way of generating human life that fails completely to respect the 'language of the body'. It is a way of generating life that simply refuses to acknowledge the deep human significance of the personal gift, bodily and spiritual in nature, of husband and wife to one another that is aptly expressed in the conjugal act, a personal gift that is itself fittingly crowned by the gift of new human life.

The recent *Catechism of the Catholic Church* also deals with this area. It can be seen as a summary of the position of the Catholic Church regarding aided-reproductive means. Although it does not add anything significant to *Donum Vitae* its tone is perhaps significant. IVF is dealt with under the sixth commandment and the subheading 'The gift of a child'. It states that Scripture and Catholic tradition have seen large families as a sign of God's blessing and the parents' generosity.[123] It recognises that couples who are sterile suffer greatly. Therefore it argues that 'research aimed at reducing sterility is to be encouraged, on condition that it is placed at the service of the human person, of his inalienable rights and his true and integral good according to the design and will of God'.[124] It goes on to quote exclusively from *Donum Vitae* making the point that homologous artificial insemination and fertilisation involving any married couples are morally unacceptable and that techniques which require the donation of sperm or ovum, and surrogate uteruses are gravely immoral.[125] Therefore, due to its theology of marriage, the marital relationship and procreation, the Catholic Church rules out all methods of aided-reproduction. Any intervention, such as deliberate experimentation, which leads to the destruction of the embryo is also ruled out due to its vision of the moral status of the embryo.

The recent encyclical *Evangelium Vitae* follows this tradition and states that the 'use of human embryos or fetuses as an object of experimentation constitutes a crime against their dignity as human beings which have a right to the same respect owed to a child once born, just as every person.'[126] This moral condemnation also includes procedures that exploit living human embryos and fetuses—sometimes specifically 'produced' for this purpose by in vitro fertilisation—either to be used as 'biological material' or as providers of organs or tissues for transplants in the treatment of certain diseases. The killing of innocent human creatures, even if carried out to help others, constitutes an absolutely unacceptable act.[127]

Some scholars have seen the prohibition in *Donum Vitae*, the *Catechism* and *Evangelium Vitae* as prophetic, in that they should encourage scientists and doctors to continue their research in order to improve and offer those technologies that could serve as simple aids to conception and to the completion of the conjugal effort. In addition, scientists and doctors should study new methods for the prevention of infertility. *Donum Vitae* could also be viewed as an incentive for everyone to rediscover and reaffirm the full humanism (all the human values in every person) that is threatened by the technological myth and by the excesses of technology applied to people without respect for their humanity.[128]

Various criticisms, both within and outside the Roman Catholic community, have been levelled against *Donum Vitae*. One particular criticism concerns the question of the status of the embryo. It appears to take for granted that the embryo, even in its very earliest stage, is a human being:

> From the moment of conception, the life of every human being is to be respected in an absolute way because man is the only creature on earth that God has 'wished for himself' and the spiritual soul of each man is immediately created by God; his whole being bears the image of the Creator.[129]

According to Michael Coughlan neither of the reasons given here are reasons for treating the embryo as a human being, but rather reasons for treating human beings with 'absolute respect'. Even this is weakly supported. The scriptural text on which God's 'wishing of man for himself' is purportedly based, is on the prayer of Jesus to the Father: 'that all may be one . . . as we are one' (John 17:21–2). But to assume that 'all' here refers to 'all human beings' seems gratuitous; the prayer is surely open to a variety of interpretations, with the consequence that the text is inadequate as a basis for this teaching. Furthermore, the reference to immediate creation of the soul has no reasonable implications for the status of the embryo, for the timing of this divine act of immediate creation has long been a matter of debate, and the church has never ruled definitively on it.

Despite this acknowledgment, *Donum Vitae* makes remarks which are tantamount to foreclosing the issue. For example it states that 'the inviolability of the innocent human being's right to life "from the moment of conception until death" is a sign and requirement of the very inviolability of the person to whom the creator has given the gift of life'.[130] Coughlan, therefore, concludes that no persuasive argument has been presented for deeming the embryo a person, or even merely an individual being. On the contrary, scientific evidence would suggest that it is more appropriate to regard the early embryo as simply a structure of human cells with a range of potentials for development into one or more individual human beings.[131]

The Vatican *Declaration on Procured Abortion* recognised the problem of the relationship of scientific evidence to theology and philosophy, especially when considering the moment when the spiritual soul is infused. It states that it is not within the competence of science to decide when the soul is infused. Rather it is a philosophical problem from which our moral affirmation remains independent for two reasons:

> (i) supposing a later animation, there is still nothing less than a human life, preparing for and calling for a soul in which the nature received from parents is completed; (ii) on the other hand it suffices that this presence of the soul be probable (and one can never prove the contrary) in order that the taking of life involves accepting the risk of killing a man, not waiting for, but already in possession of his soul.[132]

Within Roman Catholic theological circles Professor Bruno Schuller, S.J, who lectures in theology at the University of Munster considers *Donum Vitae* largely to be an exhortation to those already convinced of the truth of the position being advanced, rather than as an analysis and agreement intended to be convincing to those who are sceptical. Schuller poses the question that it is possible that medical interventions may have the characteristics of love and giving which *Donum Vitae* requires in actions that are to be the source of new life. He argues that the reason for a couple's turning to technological intervention and specifically to homologous artificial insemination is not to replace or degrade sexual activity, but rather to remedy a defect in their own conjugal act, a defect which produces a *de facto* separation of intercourse and procreation.[133]

While John Haas, an American moral theologian, sees *Donum Vitae* as offering 'a reasoned expectation of basic human goods and values to be safeguarded and promoted', he stresses the contribution that the *Instruction* makes to the defence of two key values: the dignity of the human person and the dignity of procreation. Haas does not dismiss artificial interventions as immoral simply on the grounds of their artificial nature, since that would be a form of ethical naturalism. But he is profoundly distrustful of the technological transformation or replacement of coitus. *Donum Vitae* itself insists repeatedly on the need for keeping technological intervention within moral limits. Haas makes it clear that in his view Catholic theology exalts the physicality of the human body and its sexual acts.[134]

Professor Lisa Sowle Cahill argues that the major question is not whether all medical control of reproduction is immoral, but what are the proper limits and uses of technology in accomplishing reproduction. 'I see no convincing argument that homologous techniques may not be evaluated as appropriate interventions in the presence of physical abnormalities, to accomplish the unity of love and procreation in the sexually expressed relation of a couple.'[135] She continues by arguing that the procreative relationship of parent to child is undeniably a great and precious good. But it is not an absolute value, one which should be sought at any cost and through any means. It follows that the love commitment of spouses sets reasonable, human and Christian parameters in which to undertake parenthood. The partnership of spouses is the humanly appropriate context for child-bearing. Thus donor methods are morally problematic. Cahill also raises some important questions regarding the procedures and says that even within marriage, the use of technology must be judged in relation to the love and commitment of spouses and by its effects on their relationship. Is the stress of IVF, for example, proportionate to the relatively low success rate? Does IVF technology lift up procreation as a goal to the same extent as did the old ethic in which procreation was the sole motive fully justifying sex? Finally she raises an issue which is on the minds of many people. Does the expenditure of social and health care resources on a 'high tech' remedy for so few meet the test of distributive justice?[136]

Both Bruno Schuller and Lisa Sowle Cahill raise important considerations which need to be taken into account. Rather than focusing just on the technique of IVF and the possibility that it might distort the connection between the life-giving and love-giving meaning of the conjugal act, or that the child may be perceived as a product, or that it adds a different dimension to the bodily and spiritual union of procreation, they introduce a person- and couple-centred approach. For a couple who cannot conceive in the normal way and who believe, after taking into account the full implications of their intended action, that IVF will enhance and deepen their existing relationship, it should be viewed as a positive remedy of a defect in their own conjugal act. Now it becomes a means of sustaining and building their family life. Within the context of a committed loving relationship the focus of attention should then centre on whether or not the procedures and their intended outcome enhance the people involved individually and as a couple. If IVF is judged to be life-giving both in the biological and relational sense then it would be difficult not to judge it as a liberating action. However, if one of the partners or the couple find that it oppresses rather than liberates, serious moral questions would need to be asked about their decision to embark upon a course of IVF.

Protestant attitudes

Apart from the Roman Catholic Church, most other churches arrive at a favourable judgment regarding IVF. Generally they see no moral objection to IVF as a procedure, although some churches have reservations about how this procedure may actually work in practice. There is however a diversity of opinion regarding donor involvement and experimentation.

With regard to IVF the Church of England teaches that responsible use of IVF to remove the disability of childlessness within marriage does not undermine the interweaving of procreational and relational goods in general within marriage. In fact, in specific marriages, it may offer an enrichment of the marriage relationship which both partners gladly accept.[137]

The Free Church Federal Council and the British Council of Churches argue that in vitro fertilisation of a woman's ovum by her husband's sperm, and implantation of the embryo at a suitable time in her womb, in principle does not pose serious moral problems. In practice, however, 'a moral objection arises if this procedure involves unjustifiable risk to the future life and well-being of the human being conceived in this way. The risk ought not to be greater than that involved in normal processes of conception and birth.'[138]

The Baptist Union of Great Britain sees no critical moral objections to this technique, together with embryo-transfer, where the ovum and sperm of a married couple are involved. However, contrary factors would be: (a) the danger as with any genetic manipulation of treating human life as mere genetic material; and (b) the question of the cost of the process in the light of just distribution of resources. Nevertheless, it argues that in many situations these factors could be outweighed by the benefit of relieving the pain of childlessness, and the responsibility of people to co-operate with God in the enrichment of life. 'Correspondingly, there is no Christian moral objection to [artificial insemination by husband] this process.'[139]

The Church of Scotland also does not see any moral difficulty where IVF is used to relieve infertility within the husband/wife relationship. However, 'when superovulation is used to produce more embryos than will be transferred to the mother's uterus, questions arise concerning the deliberate creation of new life without hope of its potential being realised'.[140]

The Methodist Church sees 'nothing intrinsically immoral in the fertilisation of a woman's eggs by her husband's sperm in an artificial environment and then transferring the fertilised egg to the wife's uterus, where hopefully, it will develop into a normal baby'.[141]

Why is there consensus within some Christian churches on this matter, while other churches oppose it? Kevin Kelly in his book *Life and Love* gives an excellent understanding of why two different judgments are arrived at.

The starting point for determining the morality of IVF for the Protestant churches seems to hinge on their understanding of marriage. Marriage is a God-given human institution with three essential goods. These are the transmission of life in the human community, a disciplined structure of living in which the individual may grow to moral maturity, and a strong and enduring relationship between them. In short, the 'procreational', 'moral' and 'relational' goods of marriage.[142]

Since the procreation of children is one of the 'goods' of marriage, Christians should undertake to remedy childlessness in marriage. Such remedies will enable married couples to live and enjoy the fullness of their marriage in all its three goods.

These three 'goods' are not perceived as being separate from each other; in fact they are intimately related. Children are viewed as the 'fruit' of married love, which is a 'life-giving' act. As well as enabling a couple to live more fully themselves, it also has the potential to create new human beings to share their parents' love and to grow and develop themselves as a loving person. That is why the 'life-giving' role of the parents' love is not restricted to 'giving life' in the sense of 'conceiving and giving birth to a new life'. Rather, the whole process of nurturing and education is an equally essential part of 'giving life'. It is in this very full sense that the Christian view of marriage believes that the procreational and relational goods of marriage should be held together. That is why, at least in principle, it welcomes any new development which can render fertile a marriage which is deprived of the procreational good.[143]

Certain opponents of IVF in the Protestant churches have pointed to the artificiality of the procedures arguing that they may render these techniques immoral. However, the document *Choices in Childlessness* puts forward the view that when an artificial procedure remedies a natural deficiency it should be welcomed. Ethical questions need arise only if it is thought that an artificial procedure was having a dehumanising effect. If this is the case, then it is the alleged 'inhumanity' of the process that causes ethical concern, not its artificiality. Kelly points out that there will be few Christians who would disagree with the position of *Choices in Childlessness* regarding the relationship between what is 'artificial' and what is 'human'.

The document argues that the popular ethical distinction between the 'natural' and the 'unnatural' is a distinction between what is in keeping with human nature and what is not; it is not a distinction between the natural and artificial. Since human beings are by nature intelligent and creative, and the adaptation of the environment to their needs is an expression of their intelligence, human artifice, such as that developed in medical technology, is in principle ethically natural. It is a mistake to condemn some piece of medical intervention as 'unnatural' simply because it is artificial and sophisticated. On the other hand, the ethical distinction between the natural and the unnatural does recognise that there are limits beyond which human intervention ought not to go. These limits are transgressed when such intervention renders our humanity less than human. What these limits are in any specific case is a matter for moral assessment and judgment.[144] Therefore, if there is an objection to be faced regarding IVF, it will not be because it is 'artificial'; it can only be because some people consider it 'inhuman'.

Another view put forward by opponents of IVF is that it is 'inhuman' because it fails to hold together the procreational and relational 'goods' of marriage. This question of holding together the procreational and relational goods of marriage is usually discussed in the context of contraception. The Church of England and other Christian churches have argued that, even when contraceptives are used, the procreational and relational 'goods' of marriage are still held together in a loving marriage. That is because these two 'goods' inspire the couple's whole relationship. They devote themselves to each other and to their children. Consequently, it is precisely within the couple's marriage relationship itself that these two 'goods' are held together. This leads *Personal Origins* to hold 'that procreation should not occur entirely outside the loving relationship; and that the loving relationship should issue in the good of children, unless there are strong reasons to the contrary'.[145] It would be permissible for a couple to decide not to have children if it was found that there was a serious risk of a child inheriting a grave genetic defect.

However, it is not essential that this 'holding together' of the procreational and relational 'goods' of marriage be fully expressed symbolically in every single act of intercourse. Even contraceptive intercourse is still truly 'life-giving' as well as loving, since it expresses and deepens the couple's life-giving love for each other and their family.

Personal Origins sees this line of argument as relevant to its discussion of IVF. It argues that if the use of contraceptives does not violate the essential 'holding together' of the procreational and relational goods of marriage, neither does the use of artificial techniques of procreation. 'As long as such techniques are not used entirely outside the context of a loving relationship' their use can be justified. The report continues by arguing that in such cases, the technique is offered as 'an aid to the restoration of a good proper to the marriage, which through some handicap has been impeded. So it is calculated to strengthen the relational good, and the bond between the various goods which go together to make a proper Christian marriage.'[146] It is with this theological background that *Personal Origins* is able to conclude that if it is permissible for a Christian couple to plan responsibly the number and timing of their children by using contraceptives then 'they will not hesitate in situations where they are not otherwise able to have children of their own to engender children by artificial means, within the context of their own loving relationship'. The document goes on to state that 'the responsible use of IVF to remove the disability of childlessness within marriage will not threaten to undermine the interweaving of procreational and relational goods in general within marriage. In fact, in specific marriages, it may offer an enrichment of the marriage relationship.' [147]

Most Christian churches are able to accept the belief that the relational and procreational goods of marriage are adequately 'kept together' when contraceptive measures are employed to prevent particular acts of intercourse being open to procreation. This is because the holding together of the procreational and relational 'goods' is situated more essentially in the loving relationship within marriage than in the act of intercourse expressing this relationship. They are, therefore, able to accommodate an artificially produced conception as long as it is still within the confines of the marriage relationship. [148]

The Christian churches also agree that any responsible use of IVF and reproductive technology must always respect the 'goods' of marriage itself. Therefore a moral evaluation of IVF should assess the implications for the institution of marriage itself, because the upholding of marriage as a good is fundamental to the whole fabric of human society; the good of the particular marriage involved, and the welfare of prospective children.

In conclusion it can be seen that the difference between the Roman Catholic Church and the other churches lies in the insistence by the Roman Catholic Church that human procreation must not be separated from its God-given setting of marital intercourse since it is there that the inseparability of the procreational and relational 'goods' is located. To violate this inseparability is tantamount to claiming dominion over the meaning of marriage itself. The other churches agree that there is a God-given meaning to marriage. However, while they recognise the importance of the marital act as a unique and powerful expression of inter-personal love, it is the relationship of love itself rather than intercourse which is the gift from God which enables us to understand marriage. This is why some Christians are beginning to think that it might be possible for couples to live a vocation of truly life-giving and life-sharing love even when they deliberately decide to have no children in their marriage. It also explains why some Christians believe that a sound marriage based on genuine love provides the only truly essential ingredient needed for parenthood. According to this view the genetic relationship of parents to their children is of secondary importance in comparison to this.[149]

THE MORALITY OF DONOR INVOLVEMENT AND QUESTIONS OF EXPERIMENTATION

The issues considered in this section are concerned with the donors of sperm or ova or embryos and surrogate mothers or women who are prepared to carry in their womb a child which is not their own. The question of the morality of experimentation on embryos was also a serious question for the Christian churches.

With regard to the involvement of a third-party donor the Christian churches raised a number of important questions which were to direct their moral decision-making. Does the involvement of a donor make this a new form of adultery in that it offends against the exclusive marital relationship? Could the involvement of donor sperm or donor ova alienate the non-contributing partner to the extent that he or she does not perceive themselves to be the true parent of the child? Since donor involvement creates a situation of multi-parentage, is this exposing the resulting child to the danger of a major psychological crisis regarding personal identity and all the harmful consequences that could flow from this? What is the attitude of donors? Could this process foster an attitude of genetic irresponsibility on the part of donors?

The various Christian churches which will be considered approach these different questions in similar ways. But what are interesting are the different conclusions arrived at.

The Church of Scotland

The Church of Scotland, like the Roman Catholic Church, is opposed to any form of donor involvement and sees 'in AID the unwarranted intrusion of a third party in the marriage relationship, which it cannot support'.[150] Hence, it states: 'Profound as feelings associated with infertility unquestionably are, the experience of infertility should not be taken to advocate practices such as AID, embryo transfer or egg donation which imply either the introduction of a third party into the marriage relationship or treat women as merely incubators or men as disinterested donors of sperm.'[151]

Like the Roman Catholic Church it also opposes all forms of experimentation of embryos.

The Church of England

The Church of England's response to the issues of donor involvement and experimentation can be seen in two documents: *Human Fertilisation and Embryology* and *Personal Origins*. In the first report, which was published as a response to the *Warnock Report* it showed a strong majority position for accepting AID while acknowledging that it was contrary to the position previously held by the Church of England. The report argues that 'it is possible for a couple today to hold in good conscience the conviction that the semen of a third party imports nothing alien into the marriage relationship and does not adulterate it as physical union would'. Therefore, the majority of the committee agreed with the report that 'those engaging in AID are, in their own view, involved in a positive affirmation of the family' and hence AID may be regarded as an acceptable practice.[152] It is important to note that this report refers only to AID.

The document *Personal Origins*, again issued by the Board for Social Responsibility, was a much more comprehensive study on human fertilisation and embryology. While acknowledging that donor sperm or ova have some of the common characteristics of adoption and adultery the report says that gamete donation should not be equated with either. Unlike adoption, the prospective parents' decision is not about an already existing child. Theirs is a 'much more consciously responsible role'.[153] They are actually deciding to bring a child into existence. Although the child is not genetically their own as a couple, the situation is very different from adultery since 'there is no breaking of the relationship of physical fidelity and there is no real relationship with a person outside the marriage'.[154] Nevertheless, while agreeing that gamete donation at 'procreation is separated from the relationship completely, at the genetic level, even though the connection between the two is preserved at the social level'[155] they cannot agree about how morally significant this is. This disagreement highlights a number of fundamental issues which society has to grapple with. Is genetic parenthood of fundamental value? Or is the social context of proper love, respect and care in which a child is parented of greater value? How one answers these questions will determine how one views gamete donation.

The Committee was also divided on whether the introduction of a donor 'introduces an element of dominion over nature which appears unjustifiable . . . and possibly even threatening to human values',[156] while others on the Committee simply saw this as a further extension of responsible control over procreation. Dangers which could arise could easily be coped with by appropriate safeguards rather than by prohibition.

The Working Party argued, regarding donor involvement, that their fundamental concern in this matter was the preservation of the good of Christian marriage, as instituted by God himself, and for the welfare of children. They felt that detailed observation and discussion would be necessary before a judgment could be made about whether these practices threaten marriage or the true welfare of children, or conversely if they are a blessing in marriage. However, they stressed that it was important to recognise the new possibilities now open to us which have never before existed. In this situation, they point out, 'our traditions of moral thought need to be extended and re-thought. It may well be that previous ways of thinking will not be sustainable on reflection. On the other hand, we should not give up too lightly positions which have been important to generations of Christians.'[157]

However, the Working Party was in full agreement over their practical rejection of surrogate motherhood. 'In surrogate motherhood the Christian institution of the family is fundamentally endangered, and thus . . . it cannot be morally acceptable as a practice for Christians.'[158]

By 1988 the issue for the Church of England appears to have moved from a theological stance on the morality of donor involvement to an acceptance that this is now current practice. Therefore, the Board for Social Responsibility recommended the setting up of a national licensing authority to regulate research and to control infertility services. The underlying principle of its recommendations was openness and truthfulness. The Board suggested that parents should be encouraged, with the help of counselling, to share the truth with their child or children: that a record be kept of a child born of a donation and that the child should have access to this information, with the possible exception of the name of the donor. It discouraged practices which might hinder the clarity of a person's genetic origins such as sperm mixing. The Board also recommended that the needs of the donors be taken into account and that there should be counselling to help them understand their responsibilities.[159]

In addressing the question of surrogacy the 1988 document followed the rejection found in *Personal Origins* stating that all surrogacy contracts should continue to be unenforceable in law and that agreements reached should be outside the protection of the law. They went on to advocate that it should be a criminal offence for any agency, commercial or non-commercial, to promote surrogacy agreements.[160]

When the question of research on embryos was addressed in *Personal Origins* two different views emerged. The Working Party begins by demonstrating that there is disagreement on the status of the human embryo in its early development. One view holds that human life from conception is a continuum and should be afforded the status and protection given to all human beings. This view would, therefore, hold that it would be difficult to consent to any research at any stage which would involve the hurt and destruction of the embryo. The other view puts forward the argument that we have to judge when a particular life has reached a stage where it possesses the essential features of the full human being and therefore must be protected. This, they believe, occurs with the completion of the period of individualisation, about 14 days. In principle, the second viewpoint believes that research could be permitted before this stage of individualisation has been reached.[161] However, they point out that although it may not be possible to afford an embryo the same protection which is given to other human beings in the first 14 days, it could be that respect for human life demands that it be protected from activities which threaten its existence, such as experimentation. Yet there is also the view that the good which will be achieved by permitting research may be a stronger principle and therefore more important than any disrespect it may involve for human life.[162]

The Working Party now addressed the question of what ends can this research be directed towards if research is permitted in principle. Here there is general agreement that if research is permissible it is 'only permissible for the good end of seeking to resolve the problems of infertility and genetic disorder'.[163] Research for other goals, such as routine monitoring of the effects of new chemical compounds, is not acceptable. The question of where one gets the embryos to experiment upon now arises. Once again there appears to be a division within the Working Party, one group supporting the idea that embryos could be produced solely for research while the other group opposing it. *Personal Origins* seems to find an adequate compromise by stating that 'to accept the principle that it is possible to consider producing embryos for research does not necessarily mean that it is right to do it in any given set of circumstances'.[164] But what of the question concerning embryos produced to remedy infertility that are no longer needed because the problems have successfully been resolved, or spare embryos in IVF treatment? The Working Party approaches this question by arguing that it 'concerns the judgment to be made whether it is better to make use of those embryos for good ends in seeking to find ways to resolve infertility problems and problems of genetic disorder or whether it is better (or a lesser evil) to dispose of them as reverently as possible'.[165] While they agree that this is a judgment which researchers must make in consultation and with the consent of the parents involved, they are limiting this research to infertility problems and genetic disorders.

The 1988 document, *Legislation on Human Infertility Services and Embryo Research*, does not add anything significant to the approach offered in *Personal Origins*. Once again it points to the range of opinion held within the Church of England on the subject of research. But it adds the proviso that if research be permitted, it should be subject to the control of a licensing authority,[166] therefore ensuring that research will not be left solely in the hands of the scientific community, and that it is the responsibility of the whole community.

When the question of using eggs from aborted fetuses for fertilisation, possible implantation or research was raised by the licensing authority, once again a diversity of opinion emerged. The retired Bishop of Birmingham, Dr Hugh Montefiore, put forward the view that it was right to use eggs from aborted fetuses in fertility treatments 'instead of throwing the bits down the sluice'. He argued that even though he was opposed to abortion except in cases where the mother's life was endangered or the child would be grossly malformed, the life of a human being is more important than the life of a potential human being. Therefore, although he found it 'abhorrent and distasteful to use tissue in this way . . . it is even more distasteful just to sluice it away'.[167]

However Dr John Polkinghorne, a member of the General Synod, put the Church of England's official line. He argued that 'one has to consider means as well as ends'. An important consideration was how this tissue was obtained. Arising from this are two fundamental issues: one is the fact that science would be creating a person whose mother had never had a real existence, and that could be damaging psychologically. The second is the question of consent. He felt in this specific case consent to the genetic use of fetal material could not be given.[168]

The Baptist Union of Great Britain and Ireland

In the evidence submitted to the Warnock Committee by the Baptist Union of Great Britain and Ireland a clear and thorough moral consideration of donor involvement is found. It points to certain 'strong contrary factors' which Christians should consider when discussing this issue. The Baptist Union argues that the 'use of unknown sperm or ova intensifies the tendency to treat human genetic material as objects to be manipulated, and even sold commercially, rather than as the basis for personality'.[169] This they believe could lead to irresponsibility on the part of the donors, because the conception of children is thus divorced from the context of responsible relationships. While they note that this can occur in other circumstances, with donor involvement it appears to be built into the process as an inevitable element. They also point out that the use of sperm and ova 'banks' could encourage the selection of certain genetic types as 'desirable', and this could easily lead to a programme of positive eugenics. This, the Baptist Union finds, 'is offensive to Christian morality, which believes that God gives value to human life rather than man'.[170] They reject the idea that AID or egg-donation could be defined as 'adultery' or 'unfaithfulness' within Christian ethics, but argue that 'it does disturb the principle of one flesh within Christian marriage, where sexual union is understood to be the active symbol of a covenantal relationship'.[171] In the light of the above 'strong contrary factors' the conclusion drawn is: 'A Christian ethic would be likely to resist the development of AID and egg-donation as a normally available method for overcoming infertility. Supporting factors would have to be very strong indeed to outweigh the contrary ones.'[172]

The Baptist Union evidence also gives a similar list of 'strong contrary factors' against the practice of womb leasing or surrogacy; these include the effect on the mother and child.

They also point out that in the United States surrogate mothers often refuse to give up their child.[173] Consequently, womb leasing or surrogacy is rejected by the Baptist Union report as 'normally unacceptable to a Christian ethic'.

When the Baptist Union addressed the question of experimentation on the embryo they raised similar issues already raised in other church reports. They found that strong contrary features make it unlikely that a Christian ethic could approve experiments on the embryo which involved interference with it that were not directly therapeutic.[174] Yet they differentiated between what they called 'interference' and 'observing'. They thought that situations might be found where the embryo could be produced for the specific purpose of observing it which could be morally acceptable. In the conclusion of their evidence to the Warnock Committee they noted that the area of greatest moral difficulty was to do with gene replacement in germ-line cells for therapeutic purposes. They advised that these developments need to be continually assessed and monitored. However they did note that the present technique could be approved by a Christian ethic.

The Baptist Union has tended to adhere to the arguments set forth in its evidence to the Warnock Committee. This is demonstrated by various other documents and consultation papers, such as the 1986 consultation paper, *Legislation on Human Infertility Services and Embryo Research.*

The Methodist Church
The Methodist Church has addressed the question of donor involvement on numerous occasions. It has continued to point out the possible difficulties which could arise concerning the relationship of the couple involved and the child. Nonetheless, it has arrived at the conclusion that 'no difference can be discerned, in principle, between donating eggs or embryos and donating sperm'. Therefore, it recommends that the welfare of the 'unborn human' should be paramount. To facilitate this it advises counselling for the couple before the procedure and afterwards for the family.[175]

When it deals with the issue of experimentation on embryos, it draws a distinction between embryos created for the specific purpose of experimentation and those which are produced in normal IVF procedures and are not implanted and can therefore be termed 'spare'. With regard to embryos created solely for research the Methodist Conference argued that any attempt to legalise the creation, for research purposes, of pre-embryos or fetuses, either by in vitro fertilisation or by natural reproduction, should be strongly opposed. The products of human conception always have human significance, and deliberately to create unborn humans as a means to an end, however worthy, is contrary, in the Working Party's view, to the Christian ethic of respect for that which is human.[176]

When the question of using 'spare' embryos which result from the IVF programme was addressed it noted that there were two grounds for opposing this research. First, the belief that the embryo was a human being with moral status and rights, and second, the slippery slope argument. Proponents of this view held that if experimentation on the embryo was allowed, then before long the medical scientists would be experimenting on babies. They feared the consequences for those involved and for society in general. However, the Methodist report held that an ethical case for permitting experiments on 'surplus' embryos, on the grounds that in this situation there is no conflict between the right to life of the individual and the good of the community, can be made. They arrive at this conclusion by arguing that a surplus pre-embryo has no prospect of any life beyond that which it already has. This otherwise wasted life is given purpose if used for experiments which might benefit humanity. They go on to state· that the pre-embryo is not an individual since 'individualisation' does not occur until the end of the pre-embryonic period, i.e. after 14 days. Therefore it cannot be known whether, if the conditions were favourable, the pre-embryo would develop into one, two or more individuals or none.[177] Yet the Working Party advises that if research work is permitted it should be controlled by an ethics committee and only permitted if there are likely to be real benefits to the human community from the knowledge gained. They rule out the creation of pre-embryos which contain living material from both humans and other species (chimaeras and hybrids); the cloning of pre-embryo cells to produce genetically identical individuals, although they state that it may be acceptable to culture one cell of a pre-embryo for diagnostic purposes while the rest is frozen. They also rule out, at the present time, the modification of an embryo's genetic constitution. This is because the pre-embryo is still part of the human community and genetic manipulation or the introduction of living material from another species would violate the humanity of the pre-embryo and the respect that is due to it. In cases of experimentation, the report stipulates that the parents of the embryos must give full and informed consent. Also the embryo should not be kept alive long enough for there to be any suggestion that individualisation could have occurred, and that after the experimentation the embryo should be disposed of reverently.[178]

The report also addressed the controversial issue of the use of human fetuses and fetal material for research and medical treatment. It argues that 'provided that a fetus has not been conceived with the intention of using it for donation or research, and has been either naturally aborted or an abortion carried out for good medical reasons, there can be no moral objection to its use to benefit others, e.g. by transplantation and related research. In principle, there is no difference between the use of aborted fetal material for research or transplantation and the use of tissue from a person recently deceased.'[179] However if fetal material is to be used in this way the following conditions should be met. The informed consent of the mother, and other with a direct involvement, is essential. This should be sought with sensitivity. The medical team caring for the mother should be separate from those involved in research or transplantation. Finally, the needs of the mother should be paramount. This means that an abortion should not be delayed for the sake of research, and should be carried out by whatever methods are in the best interest of the mother, even if these result in the aborted fetus being unusable.[180]

While the Methodist Church raises the problems of donor involvement it does not rule it out exclusively. Although it appears to favour research on 'spare' embryos it ensures that there are sufficient safeguards built into their treatment of the subject to limit research to areas which will be beneficial for infertility treatments and genetic abnormalities.

In conclusion it can be said that while no church condemns donor involvement in IVF as a form of adultery some believe that it is not really in accord with the exclusivity of the marriage covenant. The possibility of alienating the non-contributing partners is acknowledged, but it is not viewed as a major objection to the practice. The possible potential harm to the IVF child due to confusion or ambiguity about personal identity is perceived as a major negative factor; so is the possibility of genetic irresponsibility. However, there is total agreement in the rejection of surrogacy or womb-leasing. The churches feel that it violates the personal dignity of the women involved and might also have harmful effects on the child.

According to Kevin Kelly no church is in unreserved favour of IVF with donor involvement. The Roman Catholic Church and the Church of Scotland are quite definite in their rejection of it. The Baptist Union is less absolute in their judgment against it. The Church of England and the Methodist Church demonstrate the divisions, on this issue, within their communities.[181] Similar positions can be found regarding experimentation on embryos. While some churches rule it out completely, others, like the Methodist Church, advise that research should be only undertaken upon 'spare' embryos and lay down strict guidelines regarding how this research is to be directed.

This survey of the different Christian approaches to the questions raised by in vitro fertilisation demonstrates that within the Christian community there is a diversity of opinion on substantial issues. While this could be perceived as a debilitating factor for moral decision-making, it could, on the other hand, be understood as an important component of the process of moral decision-making in a pluralist society.

GENETICS AND ITS CHALLENGES TO MORALITY

Many commentators believe that our knowledge of human genetic make-up will transform the way we look at ourselves. Just as the discoveries of Galileo, Kepler and Copernicus humbled humanity when they dismissed the ancient anthropocentric view of the universe, so too did Darwin's revolution further reduce humanity's role in the scheme of things. Now genetic research is breaking down the code for a human being into a text of three billion chemical letters. Scientific advancement is once again necessitating a re-evaluation of the place *homo sapiens* holds in creation.[1]

Yet with these new projects there is a fear amongst people that science is running out of control. Throughout Europe, there is a massive popular demand for tight governmental controls over the applications of genetic engineering to humans. An opinion poll, published by the European Commission, found that more than 85% of all European citizens believed that their governments should intervene to regulate the new genetics. Denmark and the Netherlands were the most concerned, whereas Portugal, Italy and Spain showed the least interest.[2]

In the United States, Congress is troubled about the $3 billion research programme, the Human Genome Project, which will tease out and analyse every gene in the human blueprint. Congress wants the US Government to set up an independent commission to oversee the ethical, legal and social implications of this 15-year project. In Britain the Nuffield Council on Bioethics has called for the Government to set up a 'central co-ordinating body' to oversee genetic testing and to monitor how it is implemented in the National Health Service, insurance industry and workplace. The Council sees testing for genetic disease as the first practical issue which society will have to face. It warns against the threat of social stigma and abuse that could result from widespread genetic screening. Potential problems are envisaged as being invasions of privacy, the misuse of confidential information, and the possibilities of eugenic abuse through improvement selective breeding.

These new genetic discoveries, according to Tom Wilkie, present society with four questions: Who has the right to know what is in someone's genes? Who has the right to ownership of genetic information? Who has the right to act on genetic information? Perhaps the fourth question is the most important: Who has the right to decide the answers to the first three?[3] However, before these questions can be addressed, a brief survey needs to be made of a number of foundational issues. First, what genes actually are. Second, the reason for genetic research and the types of screening programmes already in practice; and finally, types of genetic testing envisaged for the future and their potential implications for society.

WHAT ARE GENES?

The inheritance of all our characteristics, including susceptibility to genetic diseases, is dependent on genes and chromosomes. 'A gene is the unit of heredity that determines the structure of a peptide chain, that is a string of amino acids which form the building blocks of enzymes and proteins . . . Every cell contains the genetic information to make an entire human being' and all 'this information is carried in deoxyribonucleic acid (DNA), the "spiral staircase" molecule described by Watson and Crick about thirty years ago.'[4] Genes are large molecules made up of a substance, DNA, whose double helical structure allows both copying and division. The particular sequence of individual chemical sub-units in a gene serves as a molecular code to specify the manufacture of a particular protein; an alteration (mutation) at even a single position of the DNA sequence may cause serious malfunction of the resulting protein. Modern advances in genetics are due to the ability to study DNA directly. It is estimated that approximately 75,000 different human genes exist. At present we have information on only one third of them. Genes are arranged in a fixed order on the chromosomes. Chromosomes are elongated strings of DNA and protein which occur in the nucleus of every cell in the body. Unlike genes, chromosomes can be seen through a microscope, especially when they become compact during cell division. In the normal human there are two sets of 23 chromosomes, 46 in all. One set of 23 is received from each parent. The members of 22 of the 23 pairs appear identical: these are the autosomes. The remaining pair, the sex chromosomes, differ between males and females. Female sex chromosomes are designated XX and male XY.[5]

D. J. Weatherall gives a dramatic picture of the scale of the problem posed by the science of genetics when he writes that in the past few years it has been possible to isolate human genes directly. This is no mean task considering the formidable statistics involved. In each cell in the body there is about two metres of DNA, tightly packed and coiled. Since there are approximately 3×10^{12} cells in the body, if all the DNA from one human being was joined end-to-end it would stretch to the moon and back about 8,000 times. Therefore, when embarking on a search for a single gene of, say one or two thousand bases we are looking for a needle in a molecular haystack which is about six million times the size of the needle. It is a tribute to the remarkable advances in recombinant DNA technology that such searches are now almost routinely successful.[6] It is estimated that our 23 pairs of chromosomes contain 50,000 to 100,000 genes and 3 to 3.5 billion base pairs. Scientists are eager to learn more about the structure and function of human genes and chromosomes, which, all taken together, are called the human genome. Thus researchers plan first to map the genome, then to sequence areas of special interest, and finally to sequence (or decipher the genetic letters contained in) all 3 to 3.5 billion base pairs that comprise our genome. This scientific quest has led to the setting up of the Human Genome Project. Its goals, according to Dr Francis Collins, Director of the US National Center for Human Genome Research, are to find by the year 2005 not just the location of 100,000 or so genes, but the exact sequence of their constituent chemical parts. If the human genome is an encyclopedia divided into 23 chapters (chromosome pairs), each gene 'sentence' is composed of three-letter 'words', which are in turn spelled by four molecular 'letters' called nucleotides—adenine (A), cytosine (C), guanine (G) and thymine (T).[7]

This massive project of gene mapping and sequencing will initially provide detailed knowledge about where important genes are located and how they function. The first application of this new knowledge will probably be diagnostic: tests will be developed for large numbers of diseases, and these tests will then be able to be used in newborn screening, pre-natal diagnosis and carrier screening. At the same time, however, gene mapping and sequencing may help scientists and clinicians to develop ways to correct, or at least compensate for, at least some genetic defects.[8]

WHY RESEARCH ON GENES?

An important question to be posed is: Why this massive human effort to map the human genome? Surely there are more worthwhile projects in the world which could benefit more profitably from this expertise and massive investment? According to the supporters of the Human Genome Project there are many possible benefits. For one thing, large numbers of the most serious human disorders are the result of a genetic abnormality. Pre-natal diagnosis of such disorders should be able to assist parents to decide whether or not to go ahead and have children who may or will be affected. As an example of this, genetic probes have become available for the detection of many genetic defects in the embryo such as Huntington's chorea.[9] At present pre-natal diagnosis of conditions such as Down's syndrome[10] and spina bifida are well established and, where they are detected, parents are often counselled and offered the possibility of an abortion.

The basis of genetic screening
At this stage it might prove worthwhile to survey, briefly, the scientific basis of genetic screening.[11] Traditionally, the analysis

of the genetic contribution to illness and human characteristics has been divided into three broad areas with their accompanying subdivisions First, there are disorders due to changes in single genes; these normally include Huntington's chorea, cystic fibrosis[12] and haemophilia.[13] Second, there are disorders influenced by more than one gene—polygenic disorders. The inheritance pattern is complicated because of the larger number of different genetic combinations and uncertainties about how the genes interact. Environmental factors frequently play a major part in such disorders, which are more often known as multifactorial diseases. Because of this, screening can yield results that are less clear-cut. At the same time, as our knowledge of all the environmental and genetic factors involved advances, it will become possible to identify individuals at increased risk for a disorder who could benefit from advice on how to minimise this risk. The could lead to screening for genetic predispositions to common diseases such as coronary heart disease[14] and some cancers.[15] Finally, there are chromosomal disorders. These fall into two broad categories:

1   Where an entire chromosome is added or is missing. For example in Down's syndrome there is an extra (third) copy of chromosome 21 found in the cells of affected individuals. In Turner's syndrome, one of the X chromosomes in girls is missing. This type of disorder is not inherited but occurs during conception.[16]

2   Rearrangement of chromosomal material. If this involves either net loss or gain of chromosomal material, harmful clinical effects are likely; on the other hand, if a simple exchange between chromosomes (translocation) or within them (inversion) has occurred, the chromosome make-up is 'balanced' and serious clinical effects are much less frequent.[17]

Types of genetic tests

All forms of genetic tests aim at identifying particular genetic characteristics but approach this in different ways. There are two main approaches.

1   The gene may be isolated if the product (protein) it normally produces is known. This approach was used for the genes involved with the main blood cell protein haemoglobin (important for tests involving sickle cell anaemia[18] and thalassaemias[19]).

2   The gene may be isolated if its position on a chromosome is known. This approach is increasingly successful in allowing genes to be isolated even when we know nothing about their function or what protein they normally produce. One reason for this success is that detailed genetic maps of the different chromosomes are being produced. This approach not only pinpoints the chromosome region where the gene lies, but can provide genetic markers (identifiable pieces of DNA) which lie close to the gene, and can enable an accurate test for a genetic disorder to be made even before the gene itself is isolated.

Direct genetic testing by DNA techniques differs from most other forms of medical testing in several important respects. Any body tissue can be used since genes are present in almost all cells. Since genes do not usually change during life, a DNA test can be performed at any time from conception onwards. This is a practical advantage for tests in early pregnancy, as it can allow the detection of a serious genetic abnormality that would not show itself until after the child is born. However, this raises difficult ethical problems, especially in relation to diseases which do not appear until later childhood or adult life.

An important discovery has been that many stretches of normal DNA vary between different people and together provide a pattern that is unique for every individual (apart from identical twins). This powerful technique, known as genetic fingerprinting, has many applications, especially in legal and criminal cases. Genetic fingerprinting also raises important ethical issues. Many people fear that if this is advocated by governments it could lead to an invasion of privacy. If this type of system comes into being strict controls will need to be kept on who has access to this information, and what it is used for.

A quite different but very important technique of genetic

testing is ultrasound imaging, which gives a virtually risk-free method of identifying structural and some functional abnormalities which can result from genetic diseases. This technique is widely used for the detection of fetal malformations during pregnancy, of which some, but not all, are genetic in origin. Some early manifestations of serious genetic disorders that may develop in later life, such as polycystic kidney disease[20] or certain types of cardiomyopathy[21] can also be detected.[22]

CURRENT GENETIC SCREENING PROGRAMMES

Genetic screening programmes are not a new development. Since the 1960s pregnant women have been routinely tested for their rhesus blood group,[23] so that damage to babies of rhesus negative women before and after birth can be prevented. Damage to future children is prevented by ensuring that rhesus negative women are given an antibody within a few hours of delivery, miscarriage or abortion. Since 1973 it has been policy to screen all newborn babies in the United Kingdom and most other European Union countries for phenylketonuria (PKU).[24] Severe mental retardation is characteristic of this disease, but can be prevented if dietary treatment is started in the first weeks of life. These two tests have now become an accepted part of primary health care, and are essentially genetic screening programmes.

It has been proposed that genetic screening should be carried out on the following groups of people. First, a section within the entire population known to be at risk. A good example of this is the screening of newborn babies for PKU. Second, subgroups within the population where the risk is known to be concentrated. This is appropriate, for example, within the Ashkenazi Jewish population for Tay-Sachs disease, a fatal brain disease of children especially frequent in this group. Third, groups in which genetic factors may be responsible for some but not all disabilities. For example, individuals with learning difficulties could be screened in order to detect those with fragile X syndrome,[25] and thus identify the families at further genetic risk.

In the future, increased understanding of the genetic

component in common diseases may lead to proposals for screening for genetic abnormalities that confer an increased risk for the individual rather than a certainty of developing the disease: for example, screening may point to an increased risk of cancer, or diabetes, or mental disease and there may not be simple or guaranteed ways of avoiding the risk of treating the condition if it develops. It is therefore important to assess, so far as possible, the character and degree of risk, to study existing experience as it increases, and to improve understanding of the social and ethical, as well as the technical, implications of genetic screening.[26]

Ethical principles governing genetic screening programmes
The traditionally accepted principles and practice of screening for disease were set out in a World Health Organisation (WHO) report in 1968.[27] These are:
1   An important disease;
2   Known history;
3   Latent or early symptomatic state;
4   Reliable screening test available;
5   Definite possible diagnosis and available treatment;
6   Natural history improved by treatment; and
7   Cost effective.
These criteria were designed for the detection of disease. They were formulated before pre-natal diagnosis with the associated option of aborting an affected fetus was current. They are at present dated and are not entirely appropriate for genetic screening. It is therefore suggested that for genetic screening to be appropriate three goals must be identified. It should contribute to improving the health of persons who suffer from genetic disorders; and/or allow carriers for a given abnormal gene to make informed choices regarding reproduction; and it should also move towards alleviating the anxieties of families and communities faced with the prospect of serious genetic disease.[28]

Further experience of genetic screening can be expected to lead to more precise definitions of its principles and goals; but at present the prime requirement is that the target disease should be serious. In the United Kingdom the Clothier Committee on the Ethics of Gene Therapy[29] recommended that the first candidates for consideration for such treatment should be those suffering from a disorder which is life-threatening, or causes serious handicap, and for which treatment is unavailable or unsatisfactory. In the context of genetic screening the definition is likely to be much wider and it is difficult to define precisely what is serious. Furthermore the perception of seriousness may vary between societies and will vary according to treatment possibilities. Therefore it is suggested that it would be better to define what should not be included in genetic screening: these are characteristics with a genetic component, but which cannot be classed as diseases.[30]

Existing screening programmes

Screening programmes are broadly divided into four groups, depending on the timing of the testing:

1   Neonatal (in the newly born);
2   Older children;
3   Treating couples or individuals before pregnancy (adults); and
4   Antenatal (during pregnancy).

Neonatal screening

The blood spot test for PKU has not created any major ethical problems, although questions could be raised about how this information is imparted to patients and how informed consent is obtained. Likewise the test for congenital hypothyroidism,[31] does not appear to have raised any major ethical problems. This may be because both diseases are severe and can be adequately treated if detected.

Neonatal screening for sickle cell anaemia is cheap and reliable and is recommended for populations with a significant incidence of this disease. Early diagnosis of affected infants reduces childhood mortality and morbidity, and allows parents to be counselled about subsequent pregnancies. In some inner city areas in the UK, all newborns regardless of ethnic origin are now screened for sickle cell anaemia. Screening, however, does detect carriers as well as affected individuals, and thus raises ethical issues for the extended families.

Neonatal screening for cystic fibrosis (CF) by indirect testing is carried out only in certain areas and is still under evaluation. There is some, but not conclusive, evidence that neonatal identification of infants with CF may improve their prognosis, because preventive management can be started before their lungs are damaged. Parents of affected children can also be offered pre-natal diagnosis in subsequent pregnancies. Pilot neonatal screening programmes for early identification of Duchenne's muscular dystrophy[32] have been set up in the UK and several other countries.[33] These programmes vary somewhat in detail and in the manner of obtaining consent. However, the X-linked nature of this disease raises particular ethical issues in terms of implication for the extended family. Should the extended family be informed? Or more specifically should a family member who is pregnant be informed? In cases like this there is always the possibility that a decision to abort the pregnancy may be arrived at. This could be due to a fear on the part of the parents of an inability to cope with a child with special needs and the lack of familial and social support. It could also be due to medical and social pressure.

Later childhood screening

Programmes of screening for specific genetic disorders are at present in the pilot stage. In Montreal, genetic screening programmes directed at high school students have been conducted for Tay-Sachs disease, beta thalassaemia and cystic fibrosis. All three projects appear to have been well accepted. Most carriers of Tay-Sachs or beta thalassaemia claimed they would want to know the carrier status of an intended spouse; a small minority of the Tay-Sachs carriers would 'reconsider' if the prospective partner proved to be a carrier. A follow-up survey of attitudes towards screening for Tay-Sachs concluded that 'students have a very positive attitude towards genetic screening in general'.[34]

Adult screening

Screening of adults may be carried out to detect existing disease or predisposition to a disease, or may identify carriers with a reproductive genetic risk. Most pre-symptomatic testing for late onset genetic disease (for example, Huntington's chorea) is currently offered to family members at risk. General screening for such late-onset genetic diseases is increasingly becoming technically feasible, though not necessarily desirable. Screening programmes for various forms of cancer which may have a genetic basis are currently the main form of genetic screening in the adult population. Testing of the gene itself is now possible for familial adenomatous polyposis, an inherited form of colorectal cancer. It may shortly become possible to screen a sub-group of women at high risk of familial breast cancer, though at present such screening is aimed at early detection of the cancer itself. These testing programmes in families already known to be at risk may be the forerunners of future screening programmes.

The general screening of individuals who may be carriers of inherited genes is currently used only as a service to those in an ethnic group known to have a high incidence of an inherited disease, for example the haemoglobin disorders and Tay-Sachs disease. Pilot projects have been undertaken in several centres to detect carriers of cystic fibrosis in adults aged between 16 and 45 years through screening in general practice. Preliminary results suggest a high uptake when individuals are offered testing and counselling through personal contact.

Testing before pregnancy is not systematically practised to any extent in the UK. Cyprus, however, offers a good example of the practice of adult screening. There antenatal screening for thalassaemia has been almost totally superseded by premarital screening. This is due to ethical objections by religious authorities to screening during pregnancy on the grounds that it excluded most options other than termination of affected pregnancies. Interestingly the Orthodox Church in Cyprus now insists on testing as a formal prerequisite to church weddings. The certificate required merely states that the partners have been tested and appropriately advised. In this way the confidentiality of the test result is preserved and the couple can exercise an informed choice about reproduction.

Screening during pregnancy

Screening during pregnancy may be carried out on the mother, on the baby, or on both. If, through screening, a woman is found to be a carrier of a gene for a recessive disorder, her partner may be offered genetic testing in order to find out whether the couple is at risk of having an affected child. If both parents carry the gene for a recessive disorder, or if the mother carries the gene for an X-linked disorder or if either parent has the gene for a dominant disorder, then tests may be done on the developing fetus. There are several methods of obtaining samples for genetic tests on the fetus, the most common being amniocentesis[35] and chorionic villus sampling (CVS).[36]

In many countries, antenatal screening tests are carried out on all women for rhesus haemolytic disease and rubella (German measles).[37] Rubella screening was the first screening programme undertaken with the objective of offering detection and abortion of potentially affected fetuses. Severe congenital disorders can result from rubella infection during pregnancy. Both rhesus and rubella screening appear to be well accepted. Whereas the finding of a rhesus negative blood group results in preventative treatment, a positive rubella test gives rise to the need for very painful decisions: whether to abort the pregnancy or to carry it to term and face the possibility of serious congenital malformations such as blindness, deafness, heart defects and mental retardation. The emotional trauma engendered by the need to consider an abortion and decide whether or not to have one cannot not be ignored. This is a major ethical issue which applies to many screening procedures where the disease is serious and where there is no effective treatment. Informing parents of the reproductive choices places a considerable burden on them, and counselling and support will be needed whatever the decision.

Ultrasound scanning of the fetus is generally practised and

routine ultrasound may reveal congenital abnormalities, some of which may have a genetic basis. Expert fetal anomaly scanning, a specialised form of ultrasound scanning, is offered to women known to be at increased risk of having a malformed fetus because of genetic or other reasons. In addition, it is increasingly offered to all women on a routine basis, as about 70 to 80% of all severe malformations can be detected. Although the majority of women are aware of ultrasound, the amount of explanation given regarding the possibility of detecting abnormalities varies greatly, as does expertise in interpreting the results. In many areas, screening is carried out to detect neural tube defects[38] (spina bifida and anencephaly). Pilot studies of screening during pregnancy for carriers for the common disorder cystic fibrosis are currently being undertaken in a number of centres. Antenatal screening is usually offered to women in specific risk groups. Normally women over the age of 35 are offered testing by chromosome studies for the presence of Down's syndrome in the baby. Down's syndrome occurs in approximately 1 in 600 of all births; but it is much less common in children born to younger women (1 in 1,500 at age 20). Its birth incidence increases with maternal age, being about 1 in 350 at age 35, and as high as 1 in 100 at age 40. These various screening programmes may lead to a great reduction in the births of affected children. However, one cannot discount the emotional effects of the decision to abort the life of a wanted and planned pregnancy on a couple. This has to be weighed against the possible emotional effects the birth of an affected child could have on the parents and the family.[39]

IMPLICATIONS OF SCREENING AND GENE THERAPY

Having discussed the various screening techniques available and the possible positive and negative consequences these screening programmes could have on the individuals and families directly affected, we need to discuss a further question: Do people actually want this new science? What are its wider implications for society? From the evidence available the answer to the first question is relatively simple, while the second is far more complex. It has been found that people actually request genetic testing. They want to know about themselves and the possibility of having unhealthy children. A good example of this is the screening offered for thalassaemia. Before the advent of screening, parents who had discovered their carrier status with the birth of their first affected child were left in a terrible predicament. 'The only way couples could avoid having affected children was to stop having children', says Dr Bernadette Modell of University College Hospital, London. 'In poor Catholic countries, where there were no contraceptives available, that meant husbands and wives could no longer even sleep with each other. They could scarcely cuddle each other for fear it would "go too far".'[40]

However, with the advent of genetic screening for thalassaemia that position has been transformed. Not only carrier couples, but communities throughout the Mediterranean—Sardinia, mainland Italy, Greece and Cyprus, as well as immigrant communities in Britain—have taken up the service enthusiastically. When an affected fetus is found the offer of an abortion is usually accepted. As a result, the number of births of babies with thalassaemia has plummeted. In Sardinia, for example, they declined by 70% in a decade, which shows that the urge to have healthy children is an extremely powerful one. According to some commentators what has been found with regard to thalassaemia will also be demonstrated with cystic fibrosis, once a proper educational and screening programme is in place.[41]

There are some genetic ailments which raise special problems of their own, for example Huntington's chorea. Because a carrier of its deadly gene is automatically a victim, it has posed awkward, and sometimes intractable questions. Should the victim be informed of the disease? If so what type of counselling is available for the victims and their family? Of course for many people the emergence of tests has been a godsend. Individuals have found they are free of the disease in whose shadow they have lived most of their lives. And even in cases where a positive test result was given, confirmation has sometimes been viewed as preferable to constant uncertainty. The trouble is that there may be strong insistence that people with a susceptibility to this disease take a test even though the disease's unpleasant symptoms would not manifest themselves for many years. For instance, should a medical school train a physician as a neurosurgeon if it was shown he or she had the Huntington gene, since the early stages of the disease are characterised by tremors and irrational behaviour? And would the military want to train a person with the gene? The answer to these questions is probably no, which means stress for the unfortunate individual who is being coerced into taking a test that he or she would prefer having nothing to do with. But there are also family pressures to ponder. Either husbands or wives will want at-risk spouses to take the test to see if their future offspring will be affected, or older children might decide to take the test themselves as they contemplate their own marriages. In these latter cases, a positive result for a son or daughter would obviously reveal that the at-risk parent was also affected. Resolving these problems will be extremely difficult.

Most vexed of all is the question of abortion. To those who oppose termination of fetuses on ethical and religious grounds, the development of genetic screening tests causes particular anxiety. They fear that more and more pregnancies will be terminated for increasingly irrelevant reasons.[42] 'What might now be seen as a noble and altruistic wish to prevent people from leading "useless" lives, may easily take us to the day when self-preservation rules, when we belong to a society that does not want to waste its time or money on people who are going to be a burden on health services', says Mrs Nuala Scarisbrick, of the anti-abortion organisation 'Life'. 'That is the philosophy of elitism and the master race.'[43] If society decides to abort fetuses with cystic fibrosis or Duchenne's muscular dystrophy will it be creating 'a search and destroy' mentality that leads to abortions for more trivial defects—diabetes, left-handedness, or colour-blindness for example? A movement in this direction by society would definitely be a recognition of philosophical elitism. What society needs to do is establish criteria and positive assistance to ensure that all its members are fully cared for and not discriminated against, either before or after birth, because of an inherited genetic disease.

There is also the question of whether society is on a slippery slope to moral degeneracy. According to Walter Bodmer and Robin McKie this is an easy allegation to make. But they point out that there is no evidence of this happening at the moment or that it might develop. They argue that in a society which permits abortion for social and economic reasons it would be unfair to accuse parents who elect to abort a forthcoming child with blighted health, after careful, painful debate, of dragging society down to some new moral nadir. Nevertheless, constraints on some 'genetic' terminations would seem to be reasonable, particularly those concerned with screening tests for sex selection, for example. If society goes down this path it could lead to a damaging distortion of the distribution of men and women, with disastrous social consequences. However, as was noted in the previous chapter, the ethical questions involved in sex selection are more complex than just the equal distribution of the sexes.

Bodmer and McKie point out that screening for thalassaemia and sickle cell anaemia has been with us for almost a decade now, and there is not the faintest indication that it has brought society nearer to the mindless practice of eugenics. Rather, most consequences of screening have been unequivocally positive.[44] According to Professor Peter Rowley of Rochester University: 'Pre-natal diagnosis has had a "pro-life" effect for couples who previously avoided pregnancy because of a genetic risk. Now they are willing to conceive. Furthermore some couples choose pre-natal diagnosis with no thought of termination but rather to prepare for the birth of a child with special needs.'[45]

In pointing out that abortion is not the perfect option Bodmer and McKie accept that it happens to be the only effective method available at the moment for dealing with serious inherited maladies. However, in the future this is unlikely to be the case, and some ingenious alternatives are already being developed. One consists of flushing out a blastocyst, the ball of cells that forms the very early embryo. This blastocyst can then be screened and re-inserted only if genetic tests prove satisfactory, thus completely avoiding the trauma of abortion, though it does not avoid the moral issue of the termination of life. Alternatively, using in vitro fertilisation techniques, it is possible to create several embryos from sperm and eggs provided by parents, and implant only those embryos that have been screened, and cleared of the inherited ailment carried by one or both of the parents.

The underlying problem behind all the issues discussed is a simple one. Molecular biology has, in an astonishingly brief space of time, been able to pinpoint the sources of much of humanity's genetic misery, but it has yet to find the means to put them right. We know the causes, but we generally remain powerless to neutralise them, other than by carrying out abortions. However, that situation is already changing. The first tentative steps to remedy these problems, with the creation of new drugs and genetic therapy, have already been taken.[46]

According to Bodmer and McKie the future direction of new pharmaceuticals in the twenty-first century will be on the mapping and sequencing of all our genes. With the identification of the triggers of disturbed protein pathways, science should be able to develop drugs that will block them, so halting the pernicious progress of diseases, for instance in conditions such as Alzheimer's disease. Medicine should also be able to attack tumours with pinpoint precision, and correct the dreadful physical deterioration associated with immune disorders like rheumatoid arthritis.[47]

Types of genetic intervention

Human gene therapy is considered by many experts to be the future direction in which medical science should develop to correct genetic deficiencies which are discovered through the various screening techniques. As was already discussed in the previous chapter there are four categories of human gene therapy. The first category is known as somatic cell gene therapy; here a genetic defect in the somatic or body cells of a patient is corrected. Germ-line gene therapy is the second; here a genetic defect in the germ, or reproductive cells of a patient are corrected so that the offspring of the patient also inherits the corrected gene. The third category is known as enhancement genetic engineering; in this instance a gene is inserted so as to try to enhance or improve a specific characteristic, for example adding an additional growth hormone to increase height. Eugenic genetic engineering is the final category; here genes are inserted in order to try to alter or improve complex human traits that depend on a large number of genes as well as on extensive interactions with the environment; for example intelligence, personality, character.[48]

The editorial of the *Journal of Medicine and Philosophy* on 'Human germ-line engineering' gives an excellent summary of arguments in favour of and against germ-line therapy. Those in favour of germ-line engineering argue that it is needed because of medical utility. Only germ-line therapy offers a true cure of the many genetic diseases prevalent in the human population. Other interventions above the causal gene can only be palliative or symptomatic. They also argue that it is a medical necessity, in that only germ-line therapy strategies can address some genetic diseases. Prophylactic efficiency is given as another argument in favour. By preventing the transmission of diseased genes, germ-line therapy would obviate the need to perform costly and sometimes risky somatic cell gene therapy in multiple generations. They also point to requests for germ-line therapy from parents as a significant factor in favour of this therapy. Finally they stress scientific freedom, pointing out that research at developing germ-line gene therapy techniques, where pursued within the bounds of acceptable human subjects research, is protected by the scientific community's rights to free enquiry.

Those members of the scientific community and society in general who oppose germ-line therapy point to the scientific uncertainty and clinical risks involved. Germ-line therapy experiments would involve too many ineliminable and unpredictable long-term risks to the transformed subjects and their offspring to be justified. Once again the slippery slope argument is invoked. Germ-line therapy techniques would open the door to attempts to enhance human traits through germ-line interventions, which could exacerbate problems of social discrimination based on those traits. They also point to the problem of consent of future generations as a factor which must be taken into consideration. Germ-line therapy experiments would involve research with early human embryos that would have effects on their offspring, effectively placing multiple human generations in the role of unconsenting research subjects. Another important counter factor is the allocation of resources. Germ-line therapy techniques will never be cost-effective enough to merit high social priority in the face of alternative approaches to the problems. Finally those opposed to this therapy argue that it would run counter to the integrity of genetic patrimony. Germ-line gene therapy techniques would violate the rights of subsequent generations to inherit a genetic endowment that has not been intentionally modified.[49]

As can be seen from these conflicting viewpoints the controversy of the ethics of germ-line therapy is vigorously debated within philosophical circles. Writing in the Spring 1992 issue of *Science and Public Affairs*, the British philosopher Baroness Mary Warnock contemplates the acceptability of germ-line therapy not to cure disease but as a means of enhancing normal characteristics. She writes that 'if it became possible, as indeed it might, to eradicate for ever immune deficiency, in particular AIDS, through germ-line therapy, the present or immediate advantage might seem sufficiently great to outweigh the argument from ignorance (however keenly felt)'. She goes on to state that she 'would not like to rule out for ever the legitimacy of germ-line genetic manipulation at the embryonic stage'.[50]

Another British philosopher has suggested that germ-line gene therapy to enhance human traits is something devoutly to be wished for. In his book *Wonderwoman and Superman*, John Harris imagines a new breed of humans created in the laboratory with their genes reinforced so that they are immune from diseases such as AIDS, malaria and hepatitis B. In addition, he confers on his imaginary creations genes which give them better resistance than average to cancer, and which allow them to live longer but without senescence. He argues favourably for the possibility of a new breed of persons with life chances not available to us now.[51] Yet while Harris supports this conclusion with extensive moral arguments, he fails to address the most crucial questions: who will provide such enhancement services, and who will control and regulate the providers? These are central to all discussions of the applications of the new genetics and more so to the prospects of germ-line therapy.

It is evident that germ-line therapy would require a corpus of highly trained genetic surgeons and that, inevitably, such people will be in short supply. Yet they will have technical control over the future genetic composition of the human race. The future of humanity's genes has hitherto been left to the gloriously messy and random business of men and women choosing their sexual partners (not always the same thing as choosing their marriage partners). Will people be willing to surrender control of this aspect of their lives to a small elite technocracy? Baroness Warnock is aware of this problem when she observes that the real reason for the general assumption throughout Europe that germ-line intervention will be prohibited is the fear of the power of doctors. People do not like the idea that someone unknown, but certainly not themselves, will be able to exercise power over not only them but also over their children by choosing, albeit a bit at random, how they should be.[52] She then goes on to make the final point in this matter, that 'we all fear, and not without reason, that one day such power might be exercised, not by benevolent doctors, but by political tyrants who would use us for their own ends'.[53]

It is perhaps fortunate therefore that, according to Tom Wilkie, many technical obstacles remain before germ-line gene therapy is a reasonable prospect. And it is certainly not clear that germ-line therapy would actually be necessary to achieve the ends which Baroness Warnock and Professor Harris regard as desirable. If germ-line therapy becomes technically attainable, somatic gene therapy will certainly also have been perfected. Just as children today are immunised against the major infectious diseases, one could imagine children in the future undergoing a somatic gene therapy session to boost many of the characteristics which Warnock and Harris think desirable. It may be possible to achieve immunity to AIDS and to encourage longevity and resistance to cancer simply by reprogramming the DNA in stem cells of the bone marrow, for example. What would not be possible would be structural alterations, such as changing eye colour: such choices would probably require germ-line therapy. If such boosting of normal traits is ever considered desirable, it might be wiser to proceed with somatic gene therapy and study its effects, not only on the children, but on society itself, before ever making a commitment to the irrevocable step of germ-line therapy.[54]

It is important to note that a large proportion of the discussion on germ-line therapy has been confined to the scientific and ethical communities. Most major governmental reports have confined themselves almost exclusively to somatic cell gene therapy. This is mainly due to the belief that germ-line therapy is too remote a possibility to be adequately addressed. Thus the Report of the British Committee on the Ethics of Gene Therapy (the so-called *Clothier Report* 1992) states that 'because little is known about the possible consequences and hazards, and any harm to future generations would take a long time to discover and deal with, this application of gene therapy needs to be considered quite separately from somatic cell gene therapy'.[55] The same position is taken by the Australian Government. Similarly the American Congress has not yet discussed the issues of germ-line therapy. But even if germ-line gene therapy had been on the agenda, it would still 'not be given great emphasis because of its technical remoteness. Congress will become interested in germ-line therapy if its application seems imminent.'[56] Other reports are, or at least seem to be, more radical in their opposition. In 1987 the German Enquete-Kommission recommended that the Bundestag forbid germ-line interventions as being criminal acts.[57] In 1988 eleven European Medical Research Councils stated that 'germ-line therapy, for the introduction of heritable genetic modifications, is not acceptable'.[58] The French Comite National Consultatif stated in

1991 that 'any attempt to deliberately alter the genome of germ cells and any gene therapy involving the risk of such alteration are absolutely prohibited'.[59]

In conclusion it could be contended that somatic line germ cell therapy is generally viewed as therapeutic and therefore morally acceptable. Germ-line therapy, on the other hand, causes more controversy. If it can be ascertained that it is genuinely therapeutic and used to correct a serious disorder some commentators would approve of its use. However, there seems to be general agreement, by medical boards and some governmental agencies, that its use for positive enhancement is unethical.

MORAL CONSIDERATIONS REGARDING SCREENING

Thus far in our discussion we have tended to concentrate on the tests employed and have only briefly alluded to the moral implications of screening. The moral questions concerned with screening do not just involve the individual concerned, but have far wider social and economic implications for society. Issues such as consent, confidentiality, employment and insurance are all areas which could be fundamentally affected by new genetic screening techniques. The problem does not appear to lie with the test itself or its results, but rather with who has access to this information and the possible effects this information might have on a person.

Information and consent

The British Department of Health's 1990 circular, *A Guide to Consent for Examination or Treatment* states that 'patients are entitled to receive sufficient information in a way that they understand about the proposed treatments, the possible alternatives and any substantial risks, so that they can make a balanced judgment. Patients must be allowed to decide whether they will agree to the treatment, and they may refuse or withdraw consent at any time.'[60] This statement makes four points relevant to screening. First, those being screened are entitled to receive sufficient information in a way that they can understand about what is proposed. Second, they must be made aware of any substantial risks. Third, they must be given time to decide whether or not to agree to what is proposed, and finally they must be free to withdraw at any time.

People who are to undergo screening for a genetic disorder should be informed about the procedure undertaken and its possible implications. This information should inform them about the condition to which the genetic disorder may give rise, how serious is it and how variable is it in its effects, as well as what the therapeutic options are. The way in which the disorder is transmitted, i.e. dominant, recessive and sex-linked mechanisms, and the significance of carrier status should also be fully explained. Patients also need to be informed about the procedures for informing them of the results, the possible implications of the results for their future and existing children and for other family members. Pregnant women should also be warned that genetic screening may reveal unexpected and awkward information, for example about paternity. It should be made clear precisely what is being screened for at each stage of the screening process. A clear statement of what will be done with the results and with the sample should be provided, and individuals should be able to stipulate that their samples not be kept.[61]

All genetic screening programmes should be voluntary. At present, all programmes of pre-natal diagnosis and nearly all programmes of carrier screening are voluntary. However, in contrast, virtually all newborn screening programmes are mandated by state governments. The reasons for this mandatory newborn screening is that such programmes protect the helpless from serious, avoidable harm through the use of low-risk, minimally intrusive diagnostic procedures. The arguments in favour of newborn screening for treatable conditions are so strong, in fact, that the overwhelming majority of parents want such screening to be performed on their newborns.

There is a second type of mandatory programme that can be distinguished from the unconditionally-mandatory screening imposed by a state. These might be termed 'contingently mandatory'. For example, an employer might hypothetically require all applicants for employment to undergo a battery of genetic-diagnostic tests. These tests are not mandatory in the sense that anyone could decide not to apply for work in a company that has adopted such a screening policy. However, the tests would be mandatory for all applicants. Similar questions may arise if health insurance companies begin requiring batteries of genetic tests before writing individual insurance policies. The debates that currently surround drug-testing in the workplace and testing for HIV virus in a variety of settings suggests that contingency-mandatory genetic testing may become an important public-policy issue in the future.[62]

Results of genetic screening and confidentiality

What we should do with the individual genetic information that will be obtained through the Human Genome Project, and controlling its use, are some of the key issues that will have to be faced in the next few years. The natural starting point is to assume absolute confidentiality, and the right of privacy with respect to knowledge of a person's genetic make-up. Unfortunately there are sufficient exceptions to this rule to show this should not be considered a hard and fast law. For instance it may be beneficial to an individual to reveal to an employer an inherited tendency to develop allergic reactions to certain substances, so that these can be avoided in the workplace. However, this type of employment screening could easily run the risk of generating new discriminations.

Within society this makes data protection a very complex issue. It treads the fine line between the rights of an individual not to have information used to his or her disadvantage, and the value that such knowledge may have for an organisation such as a charity for fund-raising, or government for improving its health care. When considering the proposal to set up databases of DNA fingerprints strong arguments can be made to demonstrate that criminals would be far more easily apprehended and convicted if there was a central register to refer to by the police. Similarly, a DNA database of soldiers would help identify those killed in action when other forms of

identification are impossible. These are straightforward, and potentially beneficial applications. Yet it is unlikely that there would be any public consensus to implement them, because of the fears advanced by the slippery slope argument. Civil liberties groups argue that if groups in society start assembling DNA databases, in a very short time additional information will be added to these files. Eventually vast ledgers of electronic data about citizens will have been created. This could lead to a variety of abuses ranging from discrimination on various levels to the possibility of blackmail.[63]

Normally after undergoing genetic screening, or indeed any form of testing, an individual should be fully informed of the results, both positive (abnormal) for the disorder being screened for, or negative (no defect is found). Difficulties arise when the screening process yields results which are unexpected, unwanted, and have not been covered by consent. For example, a sex chromosome abnormality may be revealed when carrying out pre-natal testing for Down's syndrome, or a different inherited disease may show up on a test designed for another purpose. To fail to disclose a serious disease accidentally discovered by testing for which consent had not been explicitly given raises ethical problems. To reveal findings affecting an individual which will not have any clinical implications but which may provoke anxiety requires careful individual consideration. Sometimes information may cause distress to the family, although future decisions about having children could be seriously affected if information is concealed. Unexpected information can present ethical dilemmas for which there are no easy answers, or indeed any correct answers.

Generally the concern is not with disclosure to the individual concerned, but with others who may be affected by the information. This particularly affects families where X-linked and autosomal dominant diseases occur. The Nuffield Council on Bioethics recommends that family members should be treated as a 'unit' and less emphasis placed on individual patient autonomy. They recommend the following principles. First, that the accepted standards of the confidentiality of medical information should be followed as far as possible. Second, that where the application of such standards might result in grave damage to the interests of other family members, then the health professionals should seek to persuade the individual, if persuasion should be necessary, to allow the disclosure of the genetic information. Finally, that in exceptional circumstances, health professionals might be justified in disclosing genetic information to other family members, despite an individual's desire for confidentiality. For example, confidentiality might justifiably be broken if an individual refused to disclose information which might prevent grave damage to other family members.[64]

Yet when considering these questions it is important not to lose sight of Article 8 (1) of the *European Convention on Human Rights* which states that 'everyone has the right to respect for his private and family life, his home and his correspondence'. The right to private life, or to privacy, clearly includes the right to be protected from the unwanted publication or disclosure of intimate personal information. Admittedly there is an ongoing debate as to what constitutes privacy, but the right to privacy includes at least 'privacy of information, that is the right to determine for oneself how and to what extent information about oneself is communicated to others'.[65] The case for confidentiality in medicine must apply with equal force in the specific area of genetic screening. Individuals agreeing to be screened need to be confident that no personal information about the results will be made available to anyone other than themselves and their medical advisers without their explicit consent. Otherwise people may be reluctant to participate, with damaging implications possibly for themselves, their families and potentially other third parties. If doctors were to break the confidence relating to genetic information, this would have adverse implications for other areas relating to the care and treatment of the patient.

However, it is also important to accept that the general right to privacy and confidentiality is not unqualified. Article 8 (2) of the *European Convention on Human Rights* provides, for example, that the individual's right to personal privacy may be overridden by requirements prescribed by law introduced to protect health or morals, or the rights and freedoms of others. This acknowledgment may be particularly important in the area of genetic screening. Information gained in the course of genetic screening will have implications for other family members which could clearly affect the future conduct of their lives.[66] The claims for this information may vary. An individual may have an interest in knowing whether a partner or prospective partner is likely to suffer from, for instance, familial colon or breast cancer, or Huntington's chorea in the future. Although this interest would be understandable, it should not be seen as a right. If this were to become the case we could easily develop into a society in which certain people were discriminated against because of the possibility of late onset diseases. The right to this knowledge changes if children with a particular partner are considered. For example, a pregnant woman may legitimately want to know the result of the screening test on the father of her child if she herself has had a positive test for the cystic fibrosis or Tay-Sachs gene. A different type of problem may arise with blood relatives where non-disclosure of information might lead to an abortion, or where a relative, not informed of a high genetic risk, might unknowingly become the parent of a child with a serious genetic disorder.[67]

Employment

An aspect of genetic screening which particularly worries people is the possible effect it may have on their employment. The possibility of using this type of information is not something new. In 1938 J. Haldane wrote:

> The majority of potters do not die of bronchitis. It is quite possible that if we really understood the causation of this disease we should find out that only a fraction of potters are of a constitution which renders them liable to it. If so, we could eliminate potters' bronchitis by regulating entrants into the potters' industry who are congenitally exposed to it.[68]

It has been suggested by some commentators that Haldane's theory could be improved upon and extended; if individual genetic variation is a significant contributor to the incidence of workplace disease, and if people could be identified and steered away from workplaces in which they were particularly susceptible to exposures, then the overall burden of occupational disease could be diminished.[69] At present there are few work-related hazards known to have a genetic origin. However, with the rapid progress of scientific developments it might be possible to codify a larger number of diseases which are affected by a particular working environment.

It is also possible that employers, in addition to identifying employees who may be exposed to any particular risk arising from a particular employment may also wish to use genetic screening to exclude people who might be at risk of non-occupational diseases, which are likely to develop regardless of the working environment. The justification for this argument is that although the onset of the disease may not be caused by or exacerbated by the workplace, the development of the disease may have implications for the manner in which the work is done, and possibly also the safety of the workplace for the individual concerned as well as for fellow employees and other third parties.

At the moment many employers already request a medical examination before granting employment. Employers are now arguing that there are valid reasons why an employer might wish to use genetic tests for occupational diseases, or might wish to have access to genetic information about other diseases which may have implications for the employment relationship. The underlying principle is competition, which forces employers to take advantage of opportunities which reduce costs and improve efficiency. Employees or job applicants who could be identified as developing work-related illnesses or illness which will impair their work performance should be excluded. This arises from the theory that healthy workers cost less. Healthy workers are not absent from work, thereby lowering the costs of hiring temporary replacements, or for retraining permanent replacements. It could also mean that fewer precautions would be needed to be taken to deal with health and safety risks. Yet it should be pointed out that market forces and the drive for economic efficiency do not provide an adequate justification for any behaviour which is ethically unsound. Ethical standards are not determined only by economic considerations, which although clearly relevant, must be balanced against the needs of others as well as of the community as a whole.[70]

There are also many good reasons why genetic screening could be in employees' best interests. It would enable employees to assess their own susceptibility to occupational disease, permitting them to make free and informed choices concerning the type of employment undertaken, while giving due consideration to personal health and safety. Employees would, in principle, be empowered to avoid occupations which would increase the risk of ill health and which in the long run might be life-threatening. In this way they could protect the economic security of themselves and their families. It would also help to provide employers with information necessary for the protection of employees by indicating who needed the protection of special health and safety measures to safeguard against the increased danger of ill health.[71]

The public interest is not solely concerned with potential benefits. There is the danger that genetic screening could lead to discrimination against those with a genetic disease. Such discrimination could be based on fear, prejudice and misunderstanding or other irrational grounds unrelated to the needs of the employer, thus leading to the possibility of widespread genetic discrimination, with its attendant social and economic costs. It is important to note that in most countries there is no legal prohibition against genetic discrimination. It is to be hoped that legislation in this area will be forthcoming and not rely on reactive policies which have determined other areas of discrimination.

In the United Kingdom so far only the armed forces require employees or job applicants to undergo genetic testing. Currently those applying for aviation training in the RAF are screened for the sickle cell gene and if it is found they are considered to be unfit for duty in such occupational categories. This is primarily because of the risk of sickling on exposure to reduced atmosphere pressure or hypoxia. It can, therefore, be concluded that despite the availability, albeit limited, of genetic screening, employers have so far decided that it is not necessary or in their interests. This is in itself significant. It is perhaps also significant that employers have not been compelled to introduce such testing through the pressure of insurance companies who provide liability insurance for employers. Although it has been pointed out that employers have not introduced genetic screening they do screen for a variety of other conditions such as drugs, alcohol and HIV. Therefore, there is the strong possibility that as genetic testing becomes more available and enters the public domain it will be seriously considered by some employers.

In the USA, where health insurance is usually provided by the employer, genetic screening of employees has more serious implications. Employers who provide health insurance may seek to avoid hiring people who may be sources of higher medical bills. There is also the danger that employees with health coverage may find it impossible to change employment without losing insurance cover in whole or in part. A family's life may be restricted by the necessity of parents of a child with a genetic disorder to maintain employment in the same state and at the same job in order to have health insurance. Recent surveys conducted in the USA seem to indicate that at present there is no major demand for the genetic testing of employees, though the possibility of more widespread use in the future should not be ruled out.

Various governmental and independent agencies, like the Nuffield Council, recommend that only where it is absolutely necessary should someone be excluded from employment. Only if an illness or condition could present a serious danger to third parties should genetic screening be required by an employer. Where the concern is limited to the health of the employee, it should be a matter for the individual employee to decide whether or not to participate in the screening programme. Where an individual does participate in a screening programme, it is possible that a responsible employer may not wish to employ someone disclosed to be at risk of a condition, particularly if its onset is unpredictable, which might imperil the employee or third parties. So far as existing genetic information is concerned, this should not normally be used to exclude people from employment unless the condition had developed so as to impair efficient performance in the job. It would be particularly inappropriate to rely on this information where the risk of disease was misunderstood by the employer or where the risk did not lead to the onset of the disease. In relation to screening for late onset genetic disorders (for example, Huntington's chorea) it is important for all involved to recognise that the genetic defect is detectable from birth, but that the individual is likely only to develop the actual disease from a relatively late age, being healthy for most of his or her life. Were this to occur it should be possible for an employer to transfer the employee to other work.[72]

In its recommendations the Nuffield Council advises that testing should occur where 'there is strong evidence of a clear connection between the working environment and the development of the condition for which the screening is conducted'; also, where 'the condition in question is one which seriously endangers the health of the employee or is one in which an affected employee is likely to present a serious danger to third parties'; and finally, where 'the condition is one for which the dangers cannot be eliminated or significantly reduced by reasonable measures taken by the employer to modify or respond to the environmental risks'.[73] Medical data on (prospective) employees can be collected for two fundamentally different purposes. The first purpose is normally to see whether, given the demands of the job and his or her physical and mental capacities, the person concerned is able to perform it without risks for his or her own health and safety or that of others. The second is to assess the employee's future ability to perform the job effectively or to predict whether he or she is a 'bad risk' for an insurance scheme or other work-related benefits.[74] There is a genuine fear that the use of genetic information for the second objective—prediction of future non-job-related disability or disease, resulting in exclusion from work or at least from work-related benefits—will begin to occur.[75]

On the other hand, the use of medical information by employers to reduce the financial burden associated with non-workplace-related disability is meeting with growing opposition.[76] The 1985 Occupational Health Services recommendation to the International Labour Organisation states that health examinations of employees should not be used for discriminatory purposes or in any other matter prejudicial to their interest.[77] The Dutch Health Council in its 1989 report on genetic testing rejected the use of tests of genetic predispositions as part of job selection procedures.[78] This is in accordance with a resolution of the European Parliament of the same year, which calls for a statutory ban on the selection of workers on the basis of genetic criteria.[79]

Insurance

The subject of genetic screening in relation to insurance is not new. In 1935 R. A. Fisher addressed the International Congress of Life Assurance Medicine on the topic, noting that 'linkage groups should be sorted out, in order to trace the inheritance and predict the occurrence of other factors of greater individual importance, such as those producing insanity, various forms of mental deficiency, and other transmissible diseases'.[80] However, it is only during the past few years that molecular techniques have provided the opportunity to realise this goal.

At present much of our experience of insurance-related ethical issues comes from Huntington's chorea. This dominantly inherited disease is rare (affecting less than one person in 10,000), of late onset and can be predicted with a high level of certainty. Nevertheless, many of the issues it raises also apply to other diseases which may have a genetic basis. Insurance is unlikely to create any new ethical issues in connection with genetic disorders whose symptoms are already manifest at the time of application. Standard insurance application forms have for many years asked about recent medical treatment as well as relevant elements of family history. Insurance companies already require applicants to give consent to the companies' access to medical records. These records may now, and will increasingly in the future, include the results of genetic screening. New ethical issues are most likely to arise as testing for late onset disorders becomes more widespread, and as genetic screening increasingly identifies individuals with a predisposition to develop certain diseases, though they will not necessarily know of any relevant family history.[81]

But it is important to note that a genetic predisposition to a disease is not always an indication of future ill health. The probability that a disease will develop can vary greatly. It may also be very difficult to predict for any given individual the age at which a disease is likely to become manifest. Any prediction is further complicated by the fact that environmental factors often play a major role in many late-onset diseases. Thus, in some cases it will be particularly difficult, if not impossible, for insurance companies to calculate the chance of an individual developing a disease, especially when little is known about its cause, and where statistical information is limited.

Although the treatment of some genetic disorders (for example cystic fibrosis) may increase their frequency in later life, treatment of others (for example phenylketonuria PKU) has removed the associated disability, while the birth incidence of many other genetic disorders amenable to genetic testing (for example, thalassaemia and Tay-Sachs disease) is falling. This is occurring because significant numbers of families have used the information made available by these tests to prevent the birth of affected children. This is normally achieved by aborting all affected children, or by a couple who run a high risk of having an affected child deciding to refrain from having children. Thus the introduction of genetic screening may actually decrease the burden to insurance companies, a factor that needs to be taken into account by the insurance industry. It is likely that in the future, as genetic screening becomes more widespread, such a reduction will continue. But this depends on encouraging the acceptance of genetic screening. This will not occur if families are penalised in insurance matters.[82]

Life insurance and health insurance are the two forms of insurance to which genetic screening is most relevant. Their relative importance varies between different societies. At present in the EU, where only a minority of individuals currently depend on private health insurance, health insurance is less important than in countries such as the USA and most other countries, where it is the principal means of paying for health care and, increasingly, has become employer based. In the future the largely American concern with health insurance in relation to genetic testing may need to be taken into account in the EU, but the need for this consideration would become serious only if there should ever be a major shift in the balance of health care costs from the public to the private sector: a development which appears to be increasingly likely when one considers the massive cutbacks that have occurred in most European national health services.

As to medical insurance, the right to health care is universally accepted.[83] The financial accessibility of health care is an essential aspect of this right. Exclusion from health insurance on the basis of genetic traits would be contrary to the right to health care, unless an alternative can be offered in the form of an adequate public coverage scheme. If there are no such schemes and health care is not provided as a freely accessible public service, private health insurance is a crucial factor in fair access to health care. In this situation, the health insurance industry inevitably becomes an instrument of social policy with the social responsibility it implies.[84] Injustice, resulting from the fact that insurance companies are merely operating on the basis of actuarial principles,[85] will increase only when more and more genetic information becomes available. That individual genetic traits should not become a basis for differential treatment as far as medical insurance is concerned, is no more than a logical consequence of the international recognition of a right to health care in the past.

For most people in the EU, life insurance is normally linked to home purchase and the covering of basic family responsibilities. It is therefore of great importance to individuals that they are not excluded from life insurance, and it is to this form of insurance that genetic screening has most relevance. The issue goes wider than the concerns of individuals. If large groups of people categorised by genetic conditions were to become effectively excluded from life insurance, then there could be serious consequences for public policy.[86]

The other area where the advent of the new genetics may have considerable adverse social consequences is that of private insurance. In general, prior to providing insurance cover for health risks, insurers will collect medical information on an individual in order to assess the magnitude of the risk. The insurers' legitimate interest to do so is recognised by the law. Requesting medical information and sometimes medical examinations also enables them to counter possible adverse selection of persons who know they are at risk from a serious disease. To the extent, however, that private insurance serves basic social needs, limitations on the insurers' freedom to collect and to use medical information in order to restrict access to coverage may be justified. Here a distinction should be made between health insurance and other private insurances, in particular life and disability insurance.[87]

As far as other forms of private insurance are concerned, the picture is more complicated. Life and disability insurance definitely have a social function, but to a lesser extent than medical insurance. Although often at least some insurance coverage for occupational disability or for loss of life must be considered as a basic social need, there is more reason here to accommodate the rights and interests of insurers on the one hand, and those of individuals seeking coverage on the other.

Nevertheless, at the international level—at least in Europe— proposals have been made which almost completely prohibit the use of genetic information by insurance companies. According to a recommendation of the Council of Europe, adopted in the beginning of 1992,[88] insurers should not have the right to require genetic testing or to enquire about results of previously performed tests, as a pre-condition for the conclusion or modification of an insurance contract. In its 1989 resolution on genetic testing, the Parliament of the European Community had already adopted a similar position.

At national level, the picture is much less clear. In most European countries the issue would seem either as yet un-debated, or discussions are still going on.[89] A recent German report concludes, that at this moment legislation restricting current underwriting practices is not called for.[90] Denmark is the only country known to be in the process of preparing a statutory ban on genetic testing by insurance companies.[91]

It should also be noted that the provisions in international human rights instruments, like the Articles 2 and 26 of the *International Covenant on Civil and Political Rights* prohibits discrimination on grounds such as race, sex or religion. It has been suggested that genetic status, or—rather—health or medical status could be specifically included in these articles, thus providing a further basis for more specific international measures safeguarding access to work and insurance.[92]

It is evident that unregulated genetic screening and dissemination of genetic information could have vast implications for individuals as well as for society. Unless strict criteria regarding the monitoring of genetic screening and the dissemination of information are adhered to there will be the risk of discrimination. On a personal level information acquired which is available to prospective partners or potential employers and insurers could determine the future direction of one's relationships, employment prospects and ability to purchase insurance. Collectively society could easily slip down the slope of discriminating against those whom it believes could parent children with genetic diseases, or have poor prospects for certain types of work or long-term employment. Thus a form of eugenic racism could emerge to create new and perhaps more invidious divisions of discrimination within society.

THE CHURCHES' RESPONSE TO GENETICS

There is no doubt that the study of genetics will be dominated for the next decades by the Human Genome Project in the USA, and by parallel research in other countries. How Christian theology responds to the many ethical dilemmas posed by genetics is a serious challenge for the churches.

The Christian churches have always taught that they have a responsibility as proclaimers of the 'Good News' to bring a specific Christian perspective and understanding of the meaning of human existence to bear on vitally important areas of human life and health. The churches have carried out this responsibility in a variety of ways. Fundamentally they perceive their role to be grounded in a series of foundational duties. With specific reference to the study of genetics they maintain that the churches have a duty to manifest and arouse in Christians a genuine awareness of the far-reaching implications of genetic decisions. If Christian compassion is not to be a hollow claim, those in leadership positions within the churches cannot remain uninformed or indifferent to the promises and perils which genetic diagnosis and counselling introduce. The churches have a duty to articulate as clearly as possible the fundamental human and Christian values that are at stake in the issue of genetic diagnosis and counselling. Broadly speaking these values can be defined as a Christian reverence for the transcendent meaning and dignity of every human life. The basic Christian orientation must be a respect for life coupled with a commitment to the sustaining of human life and the fostering of the development of human life. Christians should demonstrate a special sensitivity and compassion for the weak, underprivileged, defenceless or defective members of the human family. This sensitivity should extend not only to the unborn but also to the parents and counsellors in their endeavour to gather, assess and cope with the data at hand in the light of their human and Christian responsibilities.[93]

Generally the churches have approached the new genetic advances cautiously. They have grappled with the question of whether humanity should embark on this type of research. What should be done with the new knowledge gained? They have also attempted to establish guidelines on how to access the morality of these new developments.

Roman Catholic theology

The German theologian Karl Rahner in a seminal essay on 'The Problem of Genetic Manipulation' (1967) makes a decisive break, for Catholic theology, from the long tradition of reacting negatively to findings of modern biological sciences.[94] According to Rahner, natural law theology does not require a static non-evolutionary view of human nature. To resist human self-manipulation, he argued, would be 'symptomatic of a cowardly and comfortable conservatism hiding behind misunderstood Christian ideals'. The appropriate attitude for Christians should be 'cool-headedness' when addressing genetic manipulation. This is a mark of human courage which God has made possible by granting responsible freedom to seek the ultimate goals of life as humans are able to conceive them. Rahner recognised the fact that the human race has always modified the natural environment, using intelligence and skill effectively if not always wisely. Whether intentionally or not, and most likely not, people have also wrought changes in genetic characteristics and status of health through diet, medicine, environment and voluntary selective breeding. Now it has been made possible to exercise God-given freedom of choice to affect the course of humanity's evolution. In 1967 Rahner's knowledge of the future possibilities of genetic manipulation were limited, nevertheless he had enough foresight to imagine the great changes in human life genetic science was soon to make. His guiding principle was not whether or not to use the techniques of genetic science but how to discriminate between applications which are in consonance with human nature and thus beneficial and those which are detrimental.[95]

Rahner's vision was influential in determining the future direction of Catholic moral theology when it began to investigate genetic research. This openness can be seen in a recent statement by Pope John Paul II when he summarises the Catholic position on reason and scientific research. He states: 'The Church defends reason and science, in which she recognises the capacity to attain the truth . . . and likewise defends the liberty of science, in which resides its dignity as a human and personal good.'[96] Catholics hold, therefore, that it is possible, in principle, for persons of good will, through shared reasoning, to discover the good and the right. This is a conviction reflected in the natural law tradition, and expressly invoked in several recent Papal Encyclicals.[97] This position does not claim that it is easy to reach moral agreement, nor does it deny the importance of distinct, historical traditions. It asserts, however, that provided people follow the requirements of sound reason, society should be able to envisage moral truth as an attainable goal.[98]

The knowledge gained by the Genome Project could, however, lead to a number of both positive and negative consequences. There are two particularly important negative consequences which could affect humanity's understanding of human freedom. The first is 'reductionism', which assumes that the human person can be reduced fundamentally to sets of genetic structures and nothing more. The second is 'determinism', which is a mechanistic interpretation supported by scientific humanists such as Jacques Monod and E. O. Wilson.[99] Their argument is that people are, in effect, prisoners of their genes. Their behaviour, ability and personality are, they assume, determined by genetic composition, and people are capable of affecting this only to a comparatively small extent. However, these theories can be countered by the belief that human subjectivity is manifest in the actual decision to pursue a scientific enquiry.[100] Scientific enquiry cannot reduce human beings to genes and nothing more, because in the scientific inquiry itself, there always has to be present the human subject, the thinking scientist, who is researching those genes and whose activity transcends the genes he or she is researching. Second, it means that human choices cannot be simply determined, because it is evident that scientists commit themselves to pursue the goal of a complete knowledge about the genetic structure, that is a goal which does not yet exist, and so cannot determine their choice. Furthermore, they freely decide what to do with the knowledge they may gain. It is not our genes which choose to get themselves investigated, it is free human persons who choose to investigate the genes.[101]

Yet it must also be acknowledged that there are many positive gains to be attained from the Human Genome Project. It could enable us to have a more comprehensive understanding of the human being as a complex union of spirit and body. It is precisely in such research that we can see the enquiring human spirit at work, uncovering the material, bodily structures of the human being, which the spirit must then acknowledge as the physical basis of its own existence and activity. Thus science, in this case, could confirm what Catholic theology has held about the make-up of the human being. Pope John Paul II alludes to this when in 1982, in an address to biological researchers, he states that the whole human person, spirit and body, is the ultimate goal of scientific research, even if the immediate object of the sciences is the body with all its organs and tissues. He goes on to point out that the human body is not independent of the spirit, just as the spirit is not independent of the body, because of the deep unity and mutual connection that exist between one and the other. He, therefore, sees the importance of scientific research which promotes knowledge of the corporeal reality and activity for the life of the spirit.[102]

It is also hoped that a deeper understanding of the human genetic structure could provide a fuller notion of what human freedom actually is. According to classic Catholic moral theology, it is a mistake to imagine that human freedom is an absolute spontaneity, such that to be free means to be able to choose to do anything we happen to want to do. Human freedom is always a limited, conditioned freedom.[103] It is reasonable to assume that human choices are not determined by their genes, but they are certainly conditioned by them. For example, if we did not have human genes we would not be human, would not have human feelings or human brains, nor the potential for human freedom. But, on the other hand, our freedom is limited by our genes. For example, some people may be genetically disposed to be long lived or short lived; these genetic facts limit what we can choose to do with our lives. But it is the human person, and not these facts, who decides what to do with his or her life. The insights gained by genetic investigation could, it is hoped, explain more fully the complexities of human freedom.[104]

Another positive effect of genetics could result in a modification of the way in which humans perceive themselves in relation to nature. In particular, the study of genetics reveals the unity of all life. This demands that humanity accepts it is a part of nature. The ramification of this acknowledgment is that ecology now becomes a central issue for human life. This perception is demonstrated in official Roman Catholic teaching. Pope John Paul II in his encyclical *Centesimus Annus* points out that people think that they can make arbitrary use of the earth, subjecting it without restraint to their will, as though it did not have its own requisites and a prior God-given purpose. Instead of carrying out their role as a co-operator with God in the work of creation, humanity is inclined to set itself up in place of God and thus ends up provoking a rebellion on the part of nature, which is more tyrannised than governed by humanity. The Pope argues that this demonstrates a poverty of human vision. This is motivated by a desire to possess things rather than to relate them to the truth, and lacking that disinterest, unselfish and aesthetic attitude that is born of wonder in the presence of being and of the beauty which enables one to see in visible things the message of the invisible God who created them. Therefore, humanity today needs to be conscious of its duties and obligations towards future generations.[105]

The knowledge that there is a basic structure which we share with all other human beings means that we have an absolutely basic common humanity. The implications of this are far-reaching. No human can have grounds for dismissing another as non-human or essentially inferior. This awareness of a common nature, therefore, has the important function of protecting individual persons from discrimination on the basis of any individual or racial characteristics.[106] Furthermore, knowledge of our genes should enable medical science to undertake a wide range of therapeutic interventions, and thus aid in relieving suffering. For all these reasons, the knowledge provided by genetic research on the genome can be a good thing.[107]

However, there are serious ethical issues which could arise with the communication of this kind of knowledge, specially knowledge about the genetic defects of individuals. In the first place, an individual has a moral right not to be compelled to know about such defects in her or his genetic make-up, as this might well be too heavy a psychological burden. Furthermore, knowledge of this kind would come under what traditional moral theology called a 'natural secret', since it touches the physical basis of personality, and, if possessed by others, would expose the individual to exploitation and possible coercion. The *Catechism* is particularly aware of the coercion which is sometimes brought to bear on parents when a fetus is diagnosed as having some type of abnormality. It states that pre-natal diagnosis is morally licit, 'if it respects the life and integrity of the embryo and the human foetus and is directed toward its safeguarding or healing as an individual . . . It is gravely opposed to the moral law when this is done with the thought of possibly inducing an abortion, depending upon the results: a diagnosis must not be the equivalent of a death sentence.'[108] It also argues that attempts 'to influence chromosomic or genetic inheritance are not therapeutic but are aimed at producing human beings selected according to sex or other predetermined qualities. Such manipulations are contrary to the personal dignity of the human being and his integrity and identity which are unique and unrepeatable.'[109]

The recent encyclical *Evangelium Vitae* specifically addresses the morality of pre-natal diagnostic techniques. Pope John Paul II argues that when these techniques do not involve disproportionate risks for the child and the mother, and are meant to make possible early therapy or even to favour a serene and informed acceptance of the child not yet born, these techniques are morally licit. But since the possibilities of pre-natal therapy are today still limited, these techniques are often used with a eugenic intention which accepts selective abortion in order to prevent the birth of children affected by various types of abnormalities. Such an attitude, according to the Pope, is shameful and utterly reprehensible, since it presumes to measure the value of a human life only within the parameters of 'normality' and physical well-being. He believes that if this practice is allowed to continue then the way will eventually be opened to legitimising infanticide and euthanasia as well.[110]

With regard to people engaged in employment it could be argued that an employer would have a right to genetic information about an employee only in so far as that information was directly related to the employee's suitability for the particular job in question.[111] However, strict guidelines would need to be established to determine what occupations actually require this type of information.

Certain episcopal conferences have attempted to address the dangers and positive advantages of genetics. The American Bishops' Conference *Pastoral Statement of U.S. Catholic Bishops on Handicapped People* issued on 16 November 1978 demonstrated a helpful methodology. In this statement the bishops enunciate a number of principles and outline the responsibilities of the church at three levels: parish, diocesan and national. The bishops clearly state that the church's responsibility is to imitate Jesus. In his earthly ministry Jesus demonstrated a prominent concern for the handicapped.[112] They became witnesses of his ministry, in that by healing their bodies he signified the spiritual healing which he had brought to all of humanity.[113] The bishops, therefore, argue that the church, which was founded by Jesus, would be derelict in its duty if it failed to show the same attention he did to handicapped people.[114]

Many handicapped people suffer because of a genetic defect while others have become handicapped due to some accident, usually subsequent to birth. But whatever may have been the origin of their condition, their rights as human persons and as Christians are clear. Although some may feel a natural shyness or reluctance in dealing with handicapped people, these feelings must not prevent Christians from working vigorously to provide the necessary and rightfully expected assistance. It is not enough merely to affirm the rights of handicapped people, the bishops state.

> We must actively work to realise these rights in the fabric of modern society. Recognising that handicapped individuals have a claim to our respect because they are persons, because they share in the one redemption of Christ, and because they contribute to our society by their activity within it, the Church must become an advocate for and with them. It must work to increase the public's sensitivity toward the needs of handicapped people and support their rightful demand for justice. Moreover, individuals and organisations at every level within the Church should minister to handicapped persons by serving their personal and social needs.[115]

The church should endeavour to ensure that the rights of handicapped people are fully recognised and implemented in society. This would have a number of beneficial effects. It would ensure that the conscience level of society was elevated in regard to people with handicaps. Furthermore, the fear and suspicions of such persons will be diminished in the mind of the public because many handicapped persons who were once shunned as 'untouchable' will be seen as capable of leading reasonably happy and productive lives. In turn such improvement in public attitudes towards the handicapped may very well lessen the call for abortion as a 'solution' for genetically defective fetuses.[116]

Who is to undertake this genetic research and how it is to be monitored and controlled is also a serious question for theology. Authors like Hans Jonas have a very pessimistic view on whether humans actually have the wisdom and virtue to use this new-found knowledge to promote the development of persons. He argues that there is a built-in drive in technology which carries it ever onwards. In our age, society is inclined to go along with technology's headlong rush all too readily. We are driven, Jonas thinks, by a technological intoxication.[117] He calls for a new ethics of self-restraint and renunciation. Accordingly he would be very cautious about placing the Human Genome Project in the hands of such flawed beings as ourselves.[118] Fr Brian Johnstone also points out that Catholic theology would argue that humans are prone to evil and the misuse of knowledge. Therefore, the persons involved in the Genome Project need the appropriate inner resources, the patterns of inner purification and self-control that we call virtues.[119] These virtues should be love of nature, love of persons, justice to persons, justice to the community, and justice to God.[120] If we understand God as, above all, a lover of the nature he has created, we can see ourselves co-operating with God, as lovers of nature, as we ensure that by our care we develop, nurture and protect it, rather than dominate, manipulate and sometimes destroy it. The basic stimulus would be to nurture nature towards the full achievements of the possibilities it contained, while always respecting its integrity. As humans we are intimately woven into the fabric of nature, thus any nurturing of nature should also promote the growth of persons. Development, nurturing and protecting therefore become integral components of our love of persons, justice to persons, and justice to the community. Domination, manipulation and destruction are violations of these virtues. It is only within the interweaving web of the relations between love of nature and love of persons that we can be assured of justice to God.

With regard to the monitoring of these genetic developments, Catholic social teaching on the notion of the common good and justice may prove helpful. It teaches that an institution can be considered just when it is structured in such a way as to enable the full participation of all in decision-making processes.[121] Therefore the community as a whole must be enabled to participate, at least through its representatives. Richard McCormick calls for a public mechanism of ongoing deliberation, assessment of progress and oversight. In this the Church has both the responsibility and right to participate in the search for solutions which are fully human.[122]

Due to the obvious difficulties Catholic theology would have with the implications of certain types of genetic research, it has attempted to construct guidelines to limit and control this research. Its key starting point is respect for persons. The instruction *Donum Vitae* teaches that what is significant about the structures of human, biological nature, is that these are the structures of human persons.[123] Human biological nature has its basis in the human genome. Therefore, the human genome is morally significant in that any action upon it also touches the human person. With regards to therapeutic, genetic intervention Pope John Paul II argued that it ' . . . will be considered in principle as desirable, provided that it tends to real promotion of the personal well-being of man, without harming his integrity or worsening his life conditions'.[124] An example of this would be somatic cell gene therapy for ADA deficiency. However it should be noted that the line between normal and the abnormal, and between therapeutic and the non-therapeutic may sometimes be hard to draw. What of genetic interventions which are not strictly therapeutic? Such interventions could include interventions aimed at improving the human biological condition. The Pope does not rule out, in principle, 'interventions aimed at improving the human biological condition'.[125] However, he lays down certain criteria which must be followed if such an intervention is to be considered morally acceptable. The basis of these criteria are the identity of the human person as one of body and soul. Thus whatever affects the body, affects the spirit and with that the person. Respect for the dignity of the person is fundamental. There are three further particular criteria. First, respect for the origin of human life through procreation, involving bodily and spiritual union of the parents, joined in marriage. Second, respect for the fundamental dignity of humanity and the common biological nature which is the basis of liberty. Finally, avoidance of manipulations tending to modify the genetic 'store' and create groups of differently endowed people, thus giving rise to the danger of provoking fresh marginalisation of people in society. This third criterion would rule out modifications which lead to discrimination between classes of people.[126]

Additional criteria, some narrow, others broader, are also

offered by different Catholic theologians. It is suggested by Franz Boeckle that a Catholic theological evaluation of the Genome Project should be based on the following criteria. The Genome Project in its research, in its application and in its supporting institutions should provide instruments for the liberation of human persons from suffering. It should enable human persons to fulfil their human potential with dignity. Human persons should be facilitated to participate justly with their fellow human beings in community. Finally it should safeguard the natural basis of our existence, that is the genetic structures which are the basis of identity, freedom and common humanity.[127]

It is argued that if genetic engineering were to follow these guiding criteria then the dangers of discrimination would be lessened. However, the difficulty appears to lie in a common acceptance of criteria and in their application to specific situations.

Protestant theology

Within Protestant theological circles there is a range of opinions on this matter, ranging from the conservative to the liberal. However there is also a corpus of official statements which attempts to steer a middle road between the two extremes.

At one end of the spectrum is Professor Paul Ramsey, who for many years was seen as the doyen of American Protestant medical ethics. In an article called 'Freedom and responsibility in medical and sex ethics: A Protestant view' two themes recur. These are the absolute ethical impropriety of embryo experimentation and the accusation that in the new bioethics, the experts are 'playing God'. In this article Ramsey is mainly dealing with IVF; but the discussion is immediately relevant to the genetic sphere. In referring to IVF scientists as those who must 'mimic nature perfectly' and to in vitro fertilisation itself as 'this artificial mimicry of nature' Ramsey makes his position clear.[128] He continues his assault by stating: 'we can clearly see the extent to which human procreation has already been replaced by the idea of "manufacturing" our progeny' and that the child is perceived 'as a product of technology is to be brought forth'.[129] While Ramsey stands at one end of the spectrum Joseph Fletcher represents the other.

Joseph Fletcher, as a consequentialist, argues for genetic engineering from, for example, social needs: 'It is entirely possible, given our present increasing pollution of the human gene-pool through uncontrolled sexual reproduction, that we might have to replicate healthy people to compensate for the spread of genetic diseases and to elevate the plus factors available in ordinary reproduction.'[130] He also refutes arguments which deny this research on the basis of morality of means. It is generally accepted in ethics that humans cannot be used as means towards an end, especially in experimental medicine. However, in arguing that the embryo is not a human person Fletcher is able to discount this objection.

To give additional strength to their views Fletcher and many other theologians argue that the laboratory reproduction of human beings is no longer human procreation. For Fletcher the crux issue is the meaning of human. He claims that human beings are makers, selectors and designers and that the more rationally anything is contrived the more human it is. He points out that any attempt to set up an antimony between natural and biological reproduction on the one hand, and artificial or designed reproduction on the other, is absurd. The real difference, he asserts, is between accidental or random reproduction and rationally willed or chosen reproduction. In either case it will be biological—according to the nature of the biological process. Laboratory reproduction is radically human: it is willed, chosen, purposed and controlled, traits which, according to Fletcher, distinguish *homo sapiens* from other animals.[131]

Between these two views is the middle ground which is represented by a number of church documents.

The Report of the World Council of Churches 1979 Conference on 'Faith, Science and the Future' is strongly influenced by political perspectives of the 1970s. Thus they write:

In considering certain biological, genetic and medical manipulations of human beings . . . we must keep sharply in mind the tragic consequences suffered by many people as a result of past eugenic theories and practices. These have all too often been used by groups in power against exploited or disenfranchised minorities. . . . [Hence,] the closest scrutiny of the social and economic conditions of . . . [human genetic analysis] application will be continuously required to ensure that such technologies contribute to a just and participatory society.[132]

While accepting that as Christians we are both creatures and co-creators with God it draws a distinction between somatic and germ-line genetic engineering. 'An individual may give informed consent to a change in his own body as in body cell alteration . . . and that change is not transmitted to future generations. The individual cannot give informed consent to the genetic alteration of subsequent generations.'[133] Such decisions should be taken in a much broader social context; they cannot be just the products of contracts between scientists and subject.

Experiments with Man: Report of an Ecumenical Consultation was published by the WCC in 1969. It identifies four types of experiment:

1   Routine treatment which, with each patient, is something of an experimental venture.
2   In the course of treatment, data are collected by which existing hypotheses, methods and medicaments are checked and improved and new ones developed.
3   Fundamental clinical research not primarily directed to any immediate therapeutic benefit. But
4   there is biomedical research relating to the manipulation of genetic material. Here, the report looks into the future and remarks that the ethical considerations involved with research of this sort differ markedly from the other three types. 'Here, the investigator and society must somehow act as guarantors of the integrity of future generations by defining the limits permissible in the manipulation of the basic material of the human species.'[134]

According to Anthony Dyson 'defining the limits' of experimentation now became the recurrent theme in church documents.[135]

This is borne out in the Anglican document *Personal Origins*. Within this document differences of approach are observed. One approach welcomed the changes and showed a readiness to accept new knowledge. Another saw humans as in danger of losing any serious sense of the boundaries of natural law and of the purposes for which things are created by God. According to this approach we run the risk of overestimating human abilities and our place in relation to nature. But both approaches seek to arrive at judgments about where the moral boundaries for human action on the natural world lie. The Working Party present six principles which they believe provide the boundaries and, indeed, the avenue for proper Christian reflection and judgment on the challenges which arise from these new technologies.

The first principle refers to 'creation and "natural law"'. Since the universe has been created by God for a purpose, its basic laws provide some limit or clue to this purpose; it is right that humanity should posit and seek for 'natural law'. It follows, therefore, that in our scientific and technological culture in which the possibilities of human endeavour appear so extensive, it is important that humanity's perspective should be shaped by learning to see the world and all of its life as being under the sovereignty of God.

The 'order of nature' is given as the second principle. This accepts that there is a structure and order in nature, and implies that humanity is not free to do as it pleases, because there is a good to be aimed at, and this good is nature itself, as destined by God for realisation at the proper time. Human dominion is, therefore, envisaged as encompassing responsibility for the order of nature.

The third principle, 'human responsibility', follows easily from the second. The human race has a divinely given dominion over and responsibility for the natural order. Human beings are stewards and trustees of what God has made and maintains. Therefore, human beings cannot escape the obligation, which comes through the light of divine revelation in Jesus Christ, to reflect upon the developing knowledge of the created order nor to exercise responsibility in making decisions.

The fourth principle brings in the 'eschatological' dimension. When divine providence is reflected upon it does not just mean God preserves the world as it is; it also means that he preserves it with a view to its ultimate transformation, which is both liberation from the 'bondage to decay' and the disclosure of new and unforeseen glories. Therefore, it would be incorrect to equate this transformation with the march of science and technology. Christians could argue that the discovery of new possibilities is an aspect of God's providential care and that, whatever the judgments on particular issues, they ought not to fear new things.

The theology of the 'Kingdom of God' follows as the fifth principle. The transformation referred to above is understood as the 'Kingdom of God' which is the sovereign rule of the Creator who will vindicate and confirm his Creator's goodness. It is the same world once created that will be redeemed and glorified. It is the good once given that will be vindicated in the end. In evaluating the new goods which emerge, Christians should also look for the preservation of those goods already given.

The final principle appeals to 'Jesus Christ and the divine purpose'. The Working Party argues that our understanding of genetics must focus on the person and ministry of Jesus Christ. In particular we should be able to learn from him the worth and dignity of human life, of the depth of possibilities for human relationships and of interdependent social life.[136]

Personal Origins, like Roman Catholic theology, also attempts to refute the contention that as humans we are 'the prisoners of our genes'. It claims that the genes we are born with do not necessarily determine our life and health. Even in the limited chemical sense we are more than the sum of our genes.[137]

In 1982 the World Council of Churches issued a document entitled *Manipulating Life*.[138] It differs from the previous documents mentioned in that it puts forward the view that faith has a lot to learn from science. It also attempts to move the debate about genetics to a broader social context. Thus: 'of special concern is the reality that the inequitable distribution of power, influence and knowledge increases the possibility of the misuse of technology'.[139] Indeed, 'many of the social and ethical issues that arise in debates about genetic engineering have less to do with genetics than with broader questions of human good'.[140] While reiterating the cautious attitude of the previous documents with regard to somatic and germ-line manipulation it takes a more positive view of the potential good effects these new technologies could have in human society. It argues that 'nonetheless, changes in genes that avoid the occurrence of diseases are not necessarily made illicit merely because those changes also alter the genetic inheritance of future generations. By overcoming a deleterious gene in future beings, the beneficial effect of such changes may actually be magnified.'[141] While appearing to encourage scientific research it nevertheless feels bound to articulate some of the fears associated with these potential developments. In its acknowledgment that many religious and ethical traditions endorse some human freedom to modify or transcend nature, it poses the question as to whether germ-line manipulations of DNA directly alter the genetic foundations of the human and 'change ourselves into something less than human?'[142]

The World Council of Churches does not attempt to give any definitive answers to the questions posed. Rather the importance and influence of the document lies in its methodological approach of openness. It claims that it is no longer feasible, in these circumstances, to depend on 'precedents from the past to provide answers to questions never asked in the past'.[143] Rather human beings must search in a spirit of faith, hope and solidarity for answers to the new questions posed by genetics.

The World Council of Churches' interest in molecular biology reached its peak in 1989 at its meeting in Moscow. A study group, chaired by Archbishop John Habgood, prepared an extensive paper on biotechnology.[144] Speaking as a worldwide body, the Council shifted attention away from the concerns of genetic developments which are felt mainly, or almost exclusively, in the technologically advanced nations. It noted that the developing world also wanted to enjoy the medical benefits of genetically engineered drugs and vaccines but had a number of important fears. They feared unrestrained exploitation such as uncontrolled experimentation of human subjects where there are no regulations, and the 'dumping' of ineffectual or dangerous pharmaceuticals on poor countries.

The Council's governing body approved eleven recommendations and proposals of a practical nature. The first group of seven recommendations deals with human genetics. Here they recommend that:

1   There is a prohibition of sex selection based on pre-natal genetic testing, and warn 'against testing for other forms of involuntary social engineering'.

2   There should be resistance to 'unfair discrimination . . . in work, health care, insurance, and education' which is based upon an individual's genome.

3   They recommend 'pastoral counselling for individuals faced with difficult reproductive choices as well as personal and family decisions resulting from genetic information'.

4   They advocate a ban on 'experiments involving genetic engineering of the human germ-line at the present time' and urge 'strict control on experiments involving genetically engineered somatic cells'.

5   Likewise they want to see 'the banning of commercialised child-bearing (i.e. partial and full surrogacy) as well as the commercial sale of ova, embryos or fetal parts and sperm'.

6   They also urge that governments prohibit embryo research. If, however, embryo experimentation is agreed upon it should only be conducted under well-defined conditions.

7   The Council also recommends that the churches be kept informed 'on how new developments in reproductive technology affect families, and especially women'. The provision of pastoral counselling for those experiencing problems in using such methods is also advised.

The other four recommendations relate to animals, plants, the environment and politics. Here the Council advocates:

8   Opposing governmental patenting of genetically altered forms of animal life.
9   Urging internationally operative controls on how genetically engineered organisms may be tested, lest there be inadvertent environmental damage.
10 Advocating a worldwide ban on using genetic technology to produce chemical or biological weaponry.
11 The Council supports international consultations by scientists, governing officials and church representatives on how genetics can be used with maximal justice and benefit.

The member churches in their own ways are asked 'to take appropriate action in their own countries to draw these matters to public attention, and to help governments, scientists, universities, hospitals, and corporations to develop suitable safeguards and controls.'

Perhaps without really intending it the Council sends a very negative message. In the prologue to the statement it is asserted that 'the potential dangers as well as the potential benefits of many forms of biotechnology' are recognised. But where are the benefits actually identified? Only in the last words of (11) is a hope for benefit expressly stated. The Council counsels caution in (2), (3) and (7), where social discrimination, reproductive choices, and protection of families and women are issues. The seven other recommendations use the language of control, banning and prohibition. In terms of theology, the positive possibilities of genetic medicine, both diagnostic and therapeutic, are simply ignored as expressions of human compassion, stewardship or co-creatorship. The constructive and humane uses of laboratory and clinical research, medicines, food production are not even mentioned.[145] In deciding on this negative approach the Council runs the risk of alienating those directly involved in genetic research.

What emerges from this brief review of the Christian churches is caution with regard to the advances of genetic engineering. However, the cautious note which they strike is well worth hearing as it demonstrates that without controls genetic engineering could violate values which are fundamental to humanity. Nevertheless an over-cautious strategy could easily overlook the many positive benefits that could be gained from genetic research. What is now essential is the development of theological criteria which can resource not only the monitoring of genetic research, but also its future evolution. These criteria could use as their foundations the theological virtues of love of nature, love of persons, justice to persons, justice to the community, and justice to God. The application of these virtues will ensure that nature is developed and nurtured to achieve its true potentiality. They will also guarantee that genetic research is primarily utilised to liberate people from suffering and enhance their human potential with dignity. Research which complies with these criteria will confirm that humanity is justice towards God, nature and itself.

4

EUTHANASIA

The term 'euthanasia' comes from two Greek words—*eu*, meaning 'well', and *thanatos*, meaning 'death'—and means 'painless, happy death'. Webster's dictionary and voluntary euthanasia organisations broaden this definition to mean the 'termination of human life by painless means for the purpose of ending severe physical suffering'[1] and as a way to deal with victims of incurable disease. Its meaning now includes an interventionist act of 'mercy killing'.

This practice is not, however, something new to humanity. According to Marvin Kohl 'as long as we respect human dignity and regard kindly acts as being at least virtuous, beneficent euthanasia, or mercy killing, will be practised and remain a moral activity. For . . . our first duty is to help most where help is most needed.'[2] This sentiment was widely found in the ancient world and euthanasia was approved in cases of incurable disease by such respected authors as Pythagoras, Plato, Sophocles, Epictetus and Cicero.[3] Seneca (4 BC to AD 65), the Stoic philosopher, in his endorsement of euthanasia wrote:

> If I can choose between a death of torture and one that is simple and easy, why should I not select the latter? As I choose the ship in which I sail and the house which I shall inhabit, so I will choose the death by which I leave life. In no matter more than in death should we act according to our desire . . . Why should I endure the agonies of disease . . . when I can emancipate myself from all my torments?[4]

But until recent times advocates of euthanasia within the Christian tradition have been few in number. The major reason for this was the widespread conviction that euthanasia is prohibited by the Fifth Commandment and thus not an option that Christians may seriously consider. In short, for Christians mercy killing is murder, and murder is not a moral option. Underpinning the authority of the Fifth Commandment is the theological conviction that only God has the right to give and take life, so the act of mercy killing is viewed as an illicit exercise of what is solely a divine prerogative.[5] However, one advocate of euthanasia, the clergyman Leslie Weatherhead, has met this conviction with a provocative counter-argument. His thesis is as follows: Christians are told that death should be left to God. Yet people do not leave birth to God: they space births, prevent births and arrange births. People should, therefore, learn to become the 'lord of death as well as the master of birth'.[6] Other twentieth-century advocates of euthanasia in the Protestant and Anglican traditions include Hastings Rashdall,[7] W. R. Inge,[8] Jerry Wilson[9] and Joseph Fletcher.[10] Roman Catholics have joined their number and include Charles Curran[11] and Daniel Maguire.[12]

Although these moralists are members of the Christian community, the most zealous advocates of euthanasia are secular ethicists. Orthodox believers, whether they be Jewish, Roman Catholic or Protestant have, on the other hand, tended to be among its more persistent critics. The sympathy for euthanasia that existed in the ancient world was largely extinguished as a result of the teaching of the Christian Church. Christianity has never sanctioned the direct killing of innocent people.[13] Robert Wennberg, however, points out that euthanasia may be compatible with Christian belief. Since mercy and compassion are at the core of Christian theology as well as being core reasons for euthanasia, the Christian community should at least seriously consider euthanasia as a legal and moral possibility.[14]

In our world the question of euthanasia has been taboo for a long time on account of the shocking excesses of the euthanasia programme of the Nazi regime in Germany in 1939–41. But with the fading memory of this shock there is an increasing tendency to approve of euthanasia in desperate, hopeless cases. In 1973,

53% of the West German population pronounced themselves in favour of active euthanasia, in 1977 the number increased to 55% and in 1984 it reached 66%.[15] In the USA likewise 53% favoured euthanasia in 1973, 59% in 1977 and 64% in 1990.[16] In England and France the percentages in 1987–88 lay at 72% and 76% respectively.[17] A survey of seven EU countries indicated that over 70% of people favoured some form of voluntary euthanasia.[18] In the Netherlands where approximately 3% of all deaths are instances of either euthanasia or assisted suicide it was found that patients requested euthanasia for the following reasons: 'Loss of dignity' (mentioned in 57% of cases), 'pain' (46%), 'unworthy dying' (46%), 'dependence on others' (33%), and 'tiredness of life' (23%). Only in a minority of cases was pain given as the sole reason for requesting euthanasia.[19]

Even though these statistics would appear to favour some form of direct voluntary euthanasia they should be read in a sceptical light. The response to surveys depends, to a large extent, on how the questions are phrased and the examples provided. In the instance of euthanasia there has been a tendency to evoke an emotive response from surveys, because of the extremely emotional cases given. It is also important to point out that what the majority believes does not necessarily make for good morality. This specific point is highlighted by the present Pope in his encyclical *Evangelium Vitae*. Here he argues that morality cannot be solely based on what the majority consider and practise, but must be grounded on an objective moral law which is written in the human heart.[20]

The question as to why euthanasia now features so prominently in Western consciousness needs to be addressed. A number of reasons for this changing attitude can be suggested. Secularisation has eroded the grip of the traditional Western religious orthodoxies which condemned suicide and euthanasia. Secular reappraisals of the rights of individuals to control their own lives, including the circumstances of their own deaths, have been followed by discussions which include voluntary euthanasia and suicide as a part of an extensive list of rights to control oneself and to engage in consensual acts with willing others. The rationale for forbidding rational suicide and voluntary euthanasia has thus come under critical re-examination as a part of a general appraisal of the scope of state authority. Advocates of the 'right to die' terminology, which actually means 'the right to be killed by a physician' often refer to the principle of self-determination. Recent Appeal Court judgments in the United Kingdom appear to uphold this principle. When commenting on the rights of a patient to accept or reject treatment, Lord Justice Butler-Sloss reasoned: 'The starting point for consideration, in my view, is the right of a human being to make his own decisions and to decide whether to accept or reject treatment, the right to self-determination.' In the same case Lord Justice Hoffmann, while citing the decriminalisation of suicide in 1961, argued that a recognition of 'the principle of self-determination should in that case prevail over the sanctity of life'.

This recognition of the right of self-determination and the perceived need to limit state authority which infringes on this right has occurred at a time when medicine has succeeded, either directly or indirectly, in prolonging the lives of individuals. However, such success is often a mixed blessing. Individuals who now survive catastrophic accidents or contract severe diseases, may be faced with severe circumscription of their abilities, both physical and mental. Human bodies can be kept alive for years in the absence of whole-brain death and in the absence of consciousness. The process of dying can be extended by weeks and months. Diseases that would have killed quickly in the past now can leave individuals totally paralysed but fully alert. Though medicine may succeed in dramatically extending life, at times it does so without having secured a quality of life which is acceptable to those whose lives are prolonged. In some countries, the absence of humane care facilities for AIDS patients compels many young people to prefer active killing to inhumane dying.

This raises the question of the role of technology in medicine. If a medical intervention is likely to prolong one's life while at the same time diminishing the quality of one's life, one may be afraid to take the risk of being saved if one is exposed to the danger of being locked into an unacceptable quality of life, from which one can find no easy exit.[21] An additional point to be noted is that high technological medical care is often delivered in a fragmented form, with a different specialist called in for each organ or particular disease. Patients are aware of being in the hands of strangers who use powerful technological tools, and they are afraid that they will be treated as objects and that their desires and hopes will not be considered. This is not an irrational fear as there is evidence to support the view that certain physicians who adhere to the principle of prolonging life at any cost will, in a case of heart failure, resuscitate even entirely hopeless patients. A good example of over-zealous behaviour is Dr Karnofsky who reports that by aggressive treatment he maintained the life of a patient with cancer of the large bowel for ten months, though the patient would have died within days or weeks had nature been allowed to take its own course.[22]

Many people today, therefore, are understandably afraid that an unnecessary long and agonising process of disease and dying will be forced upon them against their will. They are afraid of a phase of lingering, harrowing sickness at the end of their lives, attached to many machines, largely immobilised, isolated and with minimal human contact.[23] In the struggle against suffering, some commentators believe that 'medicine has created new sufferings which exceed in cruelty the limits of natural sufferings'.[24] The principle of a prolongation of life at all costs raised to an absolute becomes a justification of 'cold inhumanity'.[25] Under the pretext of respect for life and duty some physicians inflict 'any torture and every humiliation' upon human beings.[26] It is therefore understandable why many people are losing hope in finding humane physicians who will help them die in a humane way.

Finally the interest in suicide, assisted suicide and voluntary euthanasia derives much of its momentum from the costs of protracted survival, particularly when prolongation of life is linked to a diminished or altogether non-existent quality of life.

Evidence indicates that 20% or more of patients who use the £1 billion invested in intensive-care units are receiving such treatment, though there is no likelihood of survival. Some of the funds could be saved simply by discontinuing treatment when it offers no benefits and only prolongs dying and suffering. Problems with medical costs are not restricted to high-intensity-care settings. The finances of retired couples and the inheritances of families are often invested in long-term nursing care which contributes little, if anything, to the quality of life of the persons receiving the care. To many, a cleaner, quicker exit may appear both more dignified, more humane and a better utilisation of resources. Therefore, there needs to be a reassessment of the moral assumptions of public policies that support the criminalisation of suicide, assisted suicide and voluntary euthanasia.[27]

Part of this reassessment has been undertaken by certain sections of the medical profession. Groups of prestigious physicians have come out in support of making lethal injections for patients legally and morally acceptable.[28] A *Boston Globe* poll claimed that 30% of physicians have no moral objections to assisting a patient to die. This change of opinion is reflected in two influential articles and attempts to legislate for euthanasia in the USA. In January 1988, the *Journal of the American Medical Association (JAMA)* published an article entitled 'It's All Over, Debbie.' This article symbolised a change in American culture toward acceptance of active euthanasia as well as being a contribution towards this change. In March 1991 the *New England Journal of Medicine (NEJOM)* followed with its own article on this issue. While the *JAMA* article had created an angry backlash, the *NEJOM* piece three years later got the same amount of media attention but very little angry criticism. In just a few years, the cultural climate for physician-administered death showed an enormous shift toward acceptance.

When the two leading medical journals in the United States endorse actively taking patients' lives and patient-assisted suicide, it can be assumed that a major cultural shift has taken place within medicine and within the broader American culture.

These shifts are normally reflected in attempts to change existing legislation. To date there have been a number of attempts to legislate for euthanasia in the United States. A legislative initiative in California called the 'Humane and Dignified Death Act', failed to get enough signatures in 1988. In Washington State, 'Initiative 119' qualified for the 1991 ballot, but was defeated at election time despite attempts on the part of its backers to confuse legalisation on assisted suicide or active euthanasia with traditional rights to refuse unwanted treatments even when they are life-sustaining.[29] In November 1994 'Measure 16' was introduced in the State of Oregon. This allows a terminally ill patient to obtain a prescription for lethal drugs from their doctor. Strict criteria apply: the patient's death must be predicted to occur within six months; there must be repeated requests from the patient and the lethal dose must be self-administered. What is now permitted is mutually assisted euthanasia.[30]

In other countries there have also been similar attempts to either legalise euthanasia or to make provision for assisted suicide. In the Netherlands where euthanasia is technically illegal the state, since the 1980s, has decided not to prosecute for direct voluntary euthanasia if certain criteria are followed. These include repeated requests by the terminally ill patient. In June 1995 the Northern Territory of Australia became the first jurisdiction in the world to allow doctors to take the lives of terminally ill patients who wish to die. Under the new Northern Territory law, an adult patient can request death, probably by a lethal injection or pill, to put an end to suffering. The patient must be diagnosed as terminally ill by two doctors, one of whom must have psychiatric qualifications. After a 'cooling off' period of seven days, the patient can sign a certificate of request. After 48 hours the wish for death can be met.

This new Northern Territory law could have a major effect on the international community. Once one country has legislated for active voluntary euthanasia it will make it easier for other countries such as Canada, the USA and certain European Community countries, which are considering introducing legislation for active voluntary euthanasia, to actually legislate for it.[31]

THE TERMINOLOGY

Certain terms have begun to emerge in our exploration into why people's attitudes towards euthanasia appear to be changing. At this juncture it is important to gain an accurate understanding of how these various terms are used and in what situations they apply.

Voluntary euthanasia

Most groups currently campaigning for changes in the law to allow euthanasia are campaigning for voluntary euthanasia—that is, euthanasia carried out at the specific request and consent of the dying person. These requests are normally made by mature, mentally competent adults who are terminally ill. Sometimes, however, voluntary euthanasia is scarcely distinguishable from assisted suicide.

Dr Jack Kevorkian,[32] a Michigan pathologist, has built a 'suicide machine' to help terminally ill people commit suicide. This machine consists of a metal pole with three different bottles attached to a tube similar to the type of tube used to provide an intravenous drip. The doctor inserts the tube into the patient's vein, but at this stage only a harmless saline solution can pass through it. The patient may then flip a switch, which will allow a coma-inducing drug to come through the tube; this is automatically followed by a lethal drug contained in the third bottle. Dr Kevorkian announced that he was prepared to make the machine available to any terminally ill patient who wished to use it. Assisting suicide is not against the law in Michigan where Dr Kevorkian initiated this practice. In the instances in which it was used where Dr Kevorkian was in attendance, he was charged with murder. However, he was acquitted as the court found that the patients had caused their own deaths.

In other cases, people wanting to die may be unable to obtain the necessary pills or even assist themselves with Kevorkian's machine. In 1973 George Zygmaniak[33] was injured in a motorcycle accident near his home in New Jersey. He was taken into hospital, where he was found to be totally paralysed from the neck down. He was also in considerable pain. He told his doctor and his brother, Lester, that he did not want to live in this condition. He begged them both to kill him. Lester questioned the doctor and hospital staff about George's prospects of recovery: he was told that they were nil. He then smuggled a gun into the hospital and shot his brother through the temple.

The Zygmaniak case appears to be a clear instance of voluntary euthanasia, although without some of the procedural safeguards that advocates of the legalisation of voluntary euthanasia propose. For instance, medical opinions about the patient's prospects for recovery were obtained only in an informal manner. Nor was there a careful attempt to establish, before independent witnesses, that George's desire for death was of a fixed and rational kind, based on the best available information about his condition. The killing was not carried out by a doctor. An injection would have been less distressing than the shooting. But these choices were not open to Lester Zygmaniak, for the law in New Jersey, as in most other places, regards mercy killing as murder and if he had made his plans known, he would not have been able to carry them out.[34]

Euthanasia can be voluntary even if a person is not actually able to cause his or her own death. That is to say, someone may, while in good health, make a written request for euthanasia if, through accident or illness, he or she becomes incapable of making or expressing a decision to die and there is no reasonable hope of recovery.[35] In killing a person who has made such a request, who has reaffirmed it from time to time, and who is now in one of the states mentioned, a physician or relative could claim to be acting with the consent of the patient.

Involuntary euthanasia
Euthanasia can be described as involuntary when the persons killed are capable of consenting to their own death but do not do so, either because they are not asked, or because when asked, choose to go on living. In the literature there appear to be very few instances of genuine involuntary euthanasia.

Non-voluntary euthanasia

There is a third category of euthanasia which is in many respects the most important. Newborn babies do not yet have, and comatose or severely brain-damaged adults have lost, the capacity to request or refuse euthanasia. In such cases neither consent nor the lack of it can be a factor. Therefore euthanasia, if considered, is neither voluntary nor involuntary, but non-voluntary.[36]

Several cases of non-voluntary euthanasia have reached the courts and the popular press. Louis Repouille[37] had a son who was described as an 'incurable imbecile', and had been bed-ridden since infancy and blind for five years. According to Repouille: 'He was just like dead all the time . . . He couldn't walk, he couldn't talk, he couldn't do anything.' In the end Repouille killed his son with chloroform.

In 1988 a case arose which demonstrates how people are forced, due to modern medical technology, to make life-and-death decisions. Samuel Linares,[38] an infant, swallowed a small object that stuck in his windpipe, causing a loss of oxygen to the brain. He was admitted to a Chicago hospital in a coma and placed on a respirator. Eight months later he was still comatose, still on the respirator, and the hospital was planning to move Samuel to a long-term care unit. Shortly before the move, Samuel's parents visited him in hospital. His mother left the room, while his father produced a pistol and told the nurse to keep away. He then disconnected Samuel from the respirator, and cradled the baby in his arms until he died. When he was sure Samuel was dead, he gave up his pistol and surrendered to police. He was charged with murder, but the grand jury refused to issue a homicide indictment, and he subsequently received a suspended sentence on a minor charge arising from the use of the pistol. Such cases raise different issues from those raised by voluntary euthanasia. In these instances there was no desire to die on the part of the infants. However it may be asked whether their deaths were carried out for the sake of the infants, or for the sake of the family as a whole.[39] What begins to emerge from these cases is the question of when death actually occurs. Louis

Repouille's son was described as 'just like dead all the time'. Do cases of this sort necessitate a re-definition of death?

DEATH

When discussing cases of non-voluntary euthanasia it is clear that there is a dispute as to when death actually occurs. Obviously the way in which society understands the time when death occurs will have an important impact on medical treatment.

To comprehend the concept of the death of a human being, it is necessary to distinguish between the definition of death, the criteria by which it can be determined that death has occurred, and the tests which show that these criteria have been satisfied. Edward Bartlett and Stuart Youngner in *Death: Beyond Whole-Brain Criteria*, argue that definitions of death are conceptual, that is, primarily abstract and philosophical. Criteria set the general physiological standards for determining whether death, as defined conceptually, has occurred. Once criteria have been determined, specific medical tests can be developed to demonstrate their fulfilment.[40]

Traditionally, the criterion for determining death was the permanent cessation of the functions of both the heart and lungs. When a person stopped breathing and his or her heart stopped beating for more than a few minutes the loss of function was irreversible and the patient was declared dead. However, the advent in recent years of new medical technology, and most importantly of respirators, has enabled modern medicine to continue by artificial means the functioning of a patient's heart and lungs after they have ceased to function naturally. In some cases heart and lung function can be restored or continued by these artificial means even after brain function has been partially or completely destroyed, for example from prolonged loss of oxygen or severe trauma to the brain. Such cases have forced a rethinking of the criteria for determination of death.[41] This has led to criteria based on whole brain and brainstem formulations, while a more extreme school of thought has developed a concept of death which resorts to a higher brain formulation.

Whole brain death

The definition of death which is based on whole brain criteria is advanced by Charles Culver and Bernard Gert,[42] the Law Reform Commission of Canada,[43] the US President's Commission on Defining Death,[44] and recently by the Danish Council of Ethics.[45]

The United States President's Commission, in its definition, states that the loss of functioning of the whole brain, either as the integrating mechanism of the body's major organ systems or as the hallmark of life itself of the human organism, is required for death. It argues that

> when all brain processes cease, the patient loses two important sets of functions. One set encompasses the integrating and co-ordinating functions, carried out principally but not exclusively by the cerebellum and brainstem. The other set includes the psychological functions which make consciousness, thought and feeling possible. These latter functions are located primarily but not exclusively in the cerebrum, especially the neocortex.[46]

ⁱThus, the whole brain formulation includes both the loss of integrating functions that make natural respiration and circulation possible, as well as the functions that make consciousness, thought and feeling possible. The Danish Council add to this understanding when they argued that death is a process and that the concept of death is bound up with the integrality of consciousness and body. ⁱThey conclude that a person should be declared dead only when all brain, heart and lung functions have definitely ceased. With the cessation of brain function, the person has entered the death process. This should not be prolonged after brain function has ceased, but that the time of death is given by the end, not the beginning of the death process. They hold that the only legitimating purpose for extending the death process is transplantation from beating heart donors, if the donor or their relatives have given their consent. In instances like this the transplant procedure will end the death process but will not constitute the cause of the donor's death.

Death, therefore, according to this understanding is 'the permanent cessation of functioning of the organism as a whole'.[47]

Brainstem death

Owing to the practical problems, particularly in transplant surgery, which arise with whole brain definitions, as pointed out in the Danish Code, an alternative theory has been sought. The search is for the physiological and anatomical core of human life, whose loss constitutes the death of the human being as a whole. There is a general acceptance that this core is identified with the brain. British medical practice employs a further identification of a physiological 'kernel' within the brain itself, namely the brainstem whose functioning underpins the functioning of the brain as a whole, hence of the human being. This theory is formidably articulated and championed by Dr Pallis[48] and David Lamb.[49] The death of the brainstem can be understood as providing the necessary and sufficient conditions for the death of the human being as a whole. Although the formal clinical diagnosis of 'brainstem death' is appropriate only under certain circumstances,[50] the death of every human being can be understood in terms of the death of the brainstem. In the vast majority of deaths, however, the formal diagnosis of brainstem death is unnecessary, since the classical cardiac diagnosis is perfectly adequate. It is in the desperate and extraordinary circumstances of the intensive-therapy unit, where a patient's underlying condition may be disguised by the artificial maintenance of their breathing and perhaps other vital functions, that greater acuity and discrimination is needed, in order to penetrate the mask of maintained functions and to diagnose the true underlying state of the unfortunate patient. If, as Pallis argues, human death is construed in terms of the final loss of brainstem function, physicians should be able to utilise diagnostic criteria with the appropriate discriminatory powers.[51]

Pallis essentially employs two arguments for the brainstem conception of death. First, the central, critical and irreplaceable characteristics of human life are functions of the brain—the brain is the 'critical system' of the human being.[52] Thus, the death of the brain as a whole implies the death of the human being. Furthermore, the brainstem is the 'critical system' within the brain. Thus the death of the brainstem implies the death of the brain as a whole. It follows, therefore, that the death of the brainstem implies the death of the human being as a whole. Second, the central, critical and irreplaceable characteristics of human life are functions of the brainstem, namely the capacities for respiration and for consciousness. The death of a human being is the irreversible loss of these capacities.[53] As can be seen, Pallis holds that the ultimate test of brainstem function is spontaneous breathing. If the brainstem is damaged by lesion or inter-cranial pressure, a coma results which is characterised by the inability to breathe spontaneously and by the absence of cranial nerve responses. This condition is irreversible.

Thus, Pallis proposes that human death is 'the irreversible loss of the capacity of consciousness combined with the irreversible loss of the capacity to breathe'.[54] These are the signs of brainstem death even though the heart may continue to beat naturally. Normally the heart will cease to function within twelve hours.[55] Pallis excludes from this definition patients with inter-cranial disorders, a coma deriving from drugs, metabolic upset, a coma following cardiac arrest, and patients in a chronic vegetative state. The vegetative state may last for months or years and has sleep/wake sequences. That is its principal difference from a coma which does not have these sequences. In the vegetative state the wake sequence is characterised by an inability to focus the eyes, to speak, or to move purposefully. Yet the automatic reactions of the eyes to light and spontaneous breathing differentiates it from an irreversible coma. This is because there is a functioning brainstem even though one or both hemispheres of the brain are damaged. He applies his definition to patients with irreversible structural brain disease caused by head injuries or inter-cranial haemorrhage. In these latter cases, if it can be shown that after two medical examinations there is an absence of brainstem reflex and a persistent inability to breathe spontaneously, the patient is dead even though the heart may continue to beat for at least twelve hours without artificial assistance.

Martyn Evans challenges this view by arguing that critics within medicine complain that some brainstem functions, above all vasomotor functions, persist, even in individuals declared 'brainstem dead' within British practice. Such persistent functions would refute, on Pallis' own terms, the notion of a dead brainstem in those individuals. By extension they would, if substantiated, refute the claim that those individuals are dead according to the brainstem criteria. Evans argues that the centrality of the brain does not exclude the vital significance of the beating heart. He goes on to point out that this redefinition of death could lead to exploitation of persistent vegetative state patients, because as things stand, the condition of the terminally comatose patient is masked by more than technology: it is masked by a diagnosis which regards the dying as already dead.[56]

Upper brain death/death of personhood

This definition, which relies on philosophical and moral criteria, defines death as the permanent absence of neo-cortical function or upper-brain death. These higher brain formulations focus exclusively on such functions as consciousness, thought and feelings which are necessary for personhood. When these have been irreversibly lost, the person is perceived to have died or permanently ceased to exist.[57] Anyone dead by the whole brain formulation will obviously be dead as well by the higher brain formulation, but not vice versa. In particular, brain injury resulting from stroke or trauma may permanently destroy all capacity for consciousness, thought and feeling, but may allow respiration and circulation to continue either assisted or unassisted. This is essentially the condition of patients in so-called persistent vegetative states who are able to breathe unaided for a number of years before death. What this concept requires is the willingness to declare as dead, persons whose circulatory and respiratory functions remain intact; that is, those whose bodies are still breathing without artificial assistance.[58]

The loss of 'personhood' as a criterion for death

Advocates of the 'higher brain death' theory like John Harris argue that when the question of what makes human life valuable is posed, the primary concern is to ascertain what makes individuals of a particular kind more valuable than others. Thus, this investigation endeavours to identify the features of particular significance which make human beings more valuable than other animals, fish and plants. These features, in turn, should point to characteristics which have moral relevance insofar as they determine why it is right to treat people as equals of one another and superiors of other creatures.

Harris, in an attempt to identify those characteristics, introduces the term 'personhood' which he defines as the capacity to want to exist and the presence of the sort of self-consciousness which makes possession of such a want possible. Where these are present, he argues, the being in whom they are present is a person. But once they are lost, the being has ceased to be a person and then, even if a body is still technically alive, it has lost its moral significance and can either be killed or allowed to die or be preserved alive. In instances where its organs or tissue can be used to save the lives of other people who have not lost their personhood but who may be in danger of losing their personhood through death or some other cause, then a motive exists for keeping alive the body of the former person so that the tissue and organs remain alive and usable.

Harris, nevertheless, recognises that there is an acute problem in determining whether or not the loss of personhood can be judged to be permanent loss, or a temporary one such that, though personhood is lost for a specific time, there may be circumstances in which the personality might return.[59] As a resolution of the problem he suggests that 'what matters is whether or not the organism is still a person, not whether or not it is dead . . . What we need, then, is not a definition of death but an account of when it is right to say that personhood is lost.'[60]

Other ethicists and moralists in their attempt to address this question of personalised death propose additional criteria for judging the presence or absence of 'personhood'. Joseph

Fletcher is generally credited with popularising the concept that the absence of brain activity means that a human person is absent. He itemises the following 'indicators of humanhood' which must be present if somebody is to be regarded as a person: they should have a minimum IQ of 40; they should be self-aware; they should be capable of exercising self-control; they should have a sense of temporal duration, a sense of the future, a sense of the past; they should be capable of entering into relationships, be capable of concern for others, be in communication with others, be in control of their existence, be inquisitive, be capable of both adapting to and initiating change in their way of life; they should enjoy a balance of reason and emotion in their life; they should be idiosyncratic or distinctive; they should have a functioning neocortex.[61] He later reduces these to four essential criteria for humanness: neo-cortical function, self-consciousness, relational ability and happiness.[62] For Fletcher the essential human trait is neo-cortical function, because behind self-consciousness and the ability to relate to others is neo-cortical life. So he holds that 'neo-cortical death means that both self-consciousness and other-orientedness are gone, whereas neither non self-consciousness nor inability to relate to others means the end of neo-cortical activity'.[63] Thus according to Fletcher's criteria, the measure of human life is a continuous personal identity while death is the loss of such a continuous identity. It follows that, according to Fletcher's criteria, a person in a persistent vegetative state is in fact in a state of death.

Other philosophers such as Robert Veatch[64] and Daniel Wikler,[65] follow a similar approach by considering the cessation of neo-cortical (upper-brain) activity to be an indication of death. This approach usually takes the following form. Death is the loss of that which is essentially significant to the nature of the entity. Consciousness (or 'the capacity to be conscious, to think, to feel, and be aware of other people') is the essentially significant characteristic of a human being. Therefore, the death of a human being is indicated by the irreversible loss of consciousness. The definition of death being proposed is the loss of that which is essentially significant (for human beings this is said to be consciousness) and the criterion for this loss is said to be irreversible upper-brain death.[66] Robert Veatch argues that what needs to be ascertained is 'when it is appropriate to treat someone as dead'.[67] And the answer Veatch gives to this question is, that this is when 'the moral claims and attributes to a living person are no longer attributed'. He thinks that moral standing disappears when a person irreversibly lacks 'an embodied capacity for consciousness or social interaction'. The oddity of Veatch's definition is highlighted by his reminder to his readers that 'when a person is dead, by definition, that person loses the right not to be killed'.[68] Veatch is distinguishing the death of the person from the death of the human being, and allowing that the person might die while the human body still lives on.

The merit of Veatch's style of argument is that it specifically focuses on persons and that when an individual permanently loses the characteristics of personhood then the obligation of other persons to care for and respect that individual also falls away.

In his analysis of this position Robert Wennberg adds an intriguing Christian perspective. He maintains that if legitimacy is granted to such a general strategy, then those operating within a Christian belief system may be attracted to the conclusion that death is the total and irreversible loss of the capacity to participate in God's creative and redemptive purposes for human life. For it is reasonable for Christians to believe that it is precisely this capacity which endows human life with its special significance. More specifically, this is the capacity to shape an eternal destiny by means of consideration of choices, soul-searching and decision-making. This requires both spiritual agency and spiritual receptivity, all of which presuppose conscious existence and not mere organic functioning. Indeed, it is reasonable to suppose that human organic life has no value in its own right but receives its significance from the fact that it can sustain personal consciousness and thereby make possible the capacity to participate in God's creative and redemptive purposes. However, when the human biological organism can no longer fulfil that function, its significance has been lost.[69]

It is possible to argue that much of the debate over how death is defined is really a covert debate about what should be done with the patient (e.g., should he or she be kept on the life-support system or disconnected from it?) and not a debate about whether the patient is really dead or not.[70] This means that Veatch's proposal that death is the irreversible loss of what is essentially significant about human life could be understood as actually being a proposal about how certain patients should be treated. Wennberg argues that these decisions must be based on an act of valuation. The fact is that conscious death can occur without organic death. This fact forces a judgment as to whether mere organic functioning without any psychological life provides a sufficient value to justify life-preserving effort. If it is agreed that human biological functioning without any conscious life (actual or potential) has no special value, then it can be claimed that the presence or absence of conscious life and not the presence or absence of organic life should be the deciding factor in deciding whether an individual is dead or allowed to die. If this cannot be agreed, then the presence or absence of organic life is the determining factor. In this case a decision is based on what is believed to be the significant characteristics of human life.

Critique of the 'personhood' definition of death

The first problem with Veatch's and similar positions is that 'death' means one thing when it is applied to human beings and another when it is applied to other animals. It therefore violates the widely accepted requirement of trans-species applicability for a definition of death.[71] For all plants and other animals death is defined as the permanent cessation of functioning of the organism as a whole. Death is a biological phenomenon and should apply equally to related species. When the death of a human being is considered it should mean the same thing as the death of a dog or a cat. This understanding is supported by ordinary usage of the term death and by law and tradition. It also accords with social and religious practices and is not likely to be affected by future changes in technology.[72]

Veatch's definition of death can also be criticised for excluding from the category of the living those human beings who are commonly considered to be alive. Examples of such are patients suffering from the permanent loss of consciousness but retaining maintenance of bodily homeostasis. This shows that it is not self-contradictory to say that a human being can be a living organism and yet have lost that which is considered to be the significant characteristic of human nature. The problem with Veatch's type of definition of death is that it describes the loss of an essentially human characteristic rather than the death of a human being. This point can be illustrated by asking: What remains after a human being has died according to Veatch's standards? Supporters of the 'essentially significant' definition hold that the loss of personhood cannot be understood as the loss of an attribute, which could be followed by death. Once it has been lost, the subsequent death is not that of a human being; instead, it is the death of a thing. They do not deny that life may go on after the person has died; rather, they assert that a human being no longer exists, and they are not concerned with the death of the organism that outlives the person.[73]

The most damaging criticism of a definition of death of Veatch's type is this: it is the definition of the loss of something essentially significant but it is not a definition of the death of the biological organism known as a human being; and furthermore, it has implications for defining death in other organisms and species. Veatch's definition may well be applied to a morally significant subset of human beings but it cannot serve as the definition of death for all human beings. The capacity to think/be conscious is not essential to the existence of a living human being. It is indeed a significant characteristic but not a necessary one and so it is imperative to look further than 'the loss of that which is essentially significant' for a definition of the death of a human being. For as John Stanley notes: the body of an upper-brain-dead (but still brainstem-alive) human being may be not only inconveniently but stubbornly alive. It may be helpless and almost totally non-sentient. It may be, ethically speaking, indistinguishable from a cadaver, but biologically speaking, it is not yet a cadaver; it is alive, and unfortunately, may remain so for some time.[74]

Owing to the imprecision of defining death according to the criteria of 'consciousness' and 'personhood', and because of the real risk involved in actually taking human life, most medical practitioners find these criteria morally indefensible. They tend to favour either the 'whole brain' or 'brainstem' criteria. Amongst Catholic moral theologians a divergence is noticed between those who are willing to accept brainstem death criteria and those who agree only to whole brain death criteria. Bernard Häring appears to favour brainstem death as it emphasises the absence of cerebral responses, induced or spontaneous movement, and an absence of spontaneous respiration.[75] George Lobo, on the other hand, demands that death should only be declared after the cessation of the integral functions of the body, thus favouring a whole brain formulation.[76] Even though many moralists and physicians reject the idea of upper-brain death, the terms which are used to define it, such as loss of personhood and loss of consciousness, have now entered the public domain. Does this imply that 'upper-brain' criteria will eventually become society's way of determining death? This has led some commentators to believe that during the 1990s the arguments to determine the criteria for death will be between the advocates of the 'whole brain' theory and the 'upper-brain' concept of death. Authors like James Drane believe that the higher-brain theorists will gain ground, but he is hopeful that resistance to this change will be met by both philosophical and non-philosophical opposition. He believes that the 'person on the street' will have something to say about this next change, and that he or she is more likely to be guided by commonsense which says that 'You aren't dead until you stop breathing.' The age-old fear of being buried alive will be enough to keep further liberalisation of brain-death legislation from occurring.[77]

THE CASE FOR EUTHANASIA

In our review of the terminology used in this discussion the arguments both for and against euthanasia have begun to emerge. As the strong counter-arguments to euthanasia will be discussed in the section dealing with the Christian churches, it is important to examine the position of the advocates of euthanasia and on what principles their arguments are founded.

The primary arguments in favour of euthanasia, whether it be voluntary or non-voluntary, appeal to the principles of compassion or mercy for the sufferer, individual self-determination or autonomy and individual well-being. Professor Flew aptly demonstrates their appeal when he writes that there are people suffering 'from incurable and painful diseases, who urgently and fixedly want to die quickly'. He says that a law which prevents this being achieved, usually forcing others to watch their pointless death helplessly, is a 'very cruel law'. He goes on to point out that such a law is very degrading in that it lacks respect for the wishes of the individual person and lacks concern for their dignity. This law evidently also demonstrates a willingness to let animal pain disintegrate the person.[78]

When discussing voluntary euthanasia it is argued that if competent patients are morally entitled to refuse any life-sustaining treatment that they judge to be sufficiently burdensome so as to make life no longer worth living with that treatment, are they not also entitled in similar circumstances to request others, such as their doctors or family members, to directly end their lives by administering a lethal injection or a poison? The same values of patient well-being and self-determination that support a patient's right to refuse any life-sustaining treatment appear to support active voluntary euthanasia.[79] Self-determination perceived as a right allows people to direct their lives in accordance with their own conception of a good life, at least within the bounds of justice and consistent with others doing so as well. In exercising this right people take responsibility for their lives and for the kinds of person they become. The implications of this view are that if rational agents autonomously choose to die, then respect for their autonomy should allow or even oblige society to assist them to do as they choose.[80]

The other main argument in support of euthanasia is individual well-being. However, it might seem that individual well-being conflicts with a person's self-determination when that person requests euthanasia. Life itself is commonly taken to be a central good for persons, often valued for its own sake, as well as necessary for pursuit of all other goods within a life. But when a competent patient decides to forgo all further life-sustaining treatment, then the patient either explicitly or implicitly decides that the best life possible for him or her with treatment is of sufficiently poor quality that it is worse than no further life at all. Life is no longer considered a benefit by the patient, but has now become a burden. The same judgment underlies a request for euthanasia: continued life is seen by the patient as no longer a benefit, but now as a burden. This phrase 'burdensome life' usually refers to the debilitated states of many critically ill or dying patients. As can be observed, in judgments of this type there are no objective standards, only the patient's own judgment as to whether continued life is no longer a benefit and has become burdensome.[81]

An appeal to mercy can also be resorted to so as to strengthen the case for active voluntary euthanasia. Consider the case of a terminally ill and imminently dying patient with a form of cancer that causes unimaginable suffering. When this competent patient implores their physician to end their suffering with a lethal poison, it seems to be cruelly perverse to hold that if a life-sustaining treatment were in place the patient's request could be honoured and death permitted, but if life-sustaining techniques were not in place a doctor could not intervene and the patient must be left to suffer in pain until nature had run its course.[82]

In terminating the lives of such patients, it is pointed out that society is not actually harming them but rather, extending mercy. This claim is supported by the fact that a natural death which cuts short an agonising dying is something people often view as a benefit and/or blessing. Death, in these circumstances, would be no less a benefit if it were brought about by direct human intervention. Therefore, those who co-operate with the terminal patient in bringing life to a close violate no one's rights; on the contrary, they perform a positive act of charity.

The final argument put forward in favour of euthanasia is that we live in a pluralist society and therefore ought not to impose our beliefs on others by means of laws whose only justification is religious in character. Accordingly, if the objection to voluntary active euthanasia is exclusively religious, then, although that may provide a good reason for members of a religious community to abstain from acts of active euthanasia, it does not provide a good reason for passing laws that prevent others who do not share those religious convictions from engaging in such acts.[83]

Involuntary euthanasia is different from voluntary euthanasia, as has been pointed out, because the person does not consent to their death, and chooses not to consent. Most ethicists believe that the rule against involuntary euthanasia is for all practical purposes absolute.

As has been noted, non-voluntary euthanasia concerns individuals who have never had the capacity to choose to live or die. This is the situation of the severely disabled infant or the older human being who has been profoundly intellectually disabled since birth, or caused to be so by accident or disease.

In the case of severely disabled infants the attitude of their parents is central to any discussion. Parents may, with good reason, regret that a disabled child was ever born. In that event, the effect that the death of the child will have on its parents can be a reason for, rather than against, killing it. The quality of life that the infant can be expected to have is also important. Peter Singer notes that when the life of an infant is so miserable as not to be worth living from the internal perspective of the being who will lead that life, and that if there are no 'extrinsic' reasons for keeping the infant alive such as the feelings of the parents, then it is better that the child should be helped to die without further suffering.[84]

Ending life without consent may also be considered in the case of those who were once persons capable of choosing to live or die, but now, through accident or old age, have permanently lost this capacity, and did not, prior to losing it, express any views about whether they wished to go on living in such circumstances.

These cases are not rare. Many hospitals care for motor accident victims whose brains have been damaged beyond all possible recovery. They may survive, in a coma, or perhaps barely conscious, for several years. In 1991, *The Lancet* reported that at any given time, between 5,000 and 10,000 Americans are surviving in a persistent vegetative state.[85] In other developed countries, where life-prolonging technology is not used so aggressively, there are far fewer long-term patients in this condition.

These human beings, according to Singer, are not self-conscious, rational or autonomous, and so considerations of a right to life or of respecting autonomy do not apply. If they have no experiences at all, and can never have any again, their lives have no intrinsic value. Life's journey has, in fact, come to an end. They are biologically alive, but not biographically. The lives of those who are not in a coma and are conscious but not self-conscious have value if such beings experience more pleasure than pain, or have preferences that can be satisfied; but it is difficult, so the argument runs, to see the point of keeping such human beings alive if their lives are, on the whole, miserable.[86]

This brief survey demonstrates that the basic principles which advocate voluntary direct euthanasia are compassion or mercy for the patient, individual self-determination and individual well-being. However when non-voluntary euthanasia is considered not only are compassion and individual well-being important factors in decision-making but also compassion for those directly concerned with the patient. In the case of infants this would be their parents, while in the case of the elderly or the persistently vegetative it would be their partners, or the broader family. It is evident that the meaning of compassion or mercy and individual well-being can vary depending on the circumstances in which people find themselves. These principles, although important, are too relative in the crucial area of life and death decisions. If an objective criterion is sought to defend euthanasia it appears that this must lie in the recognition of the right to self-determination. An acceptance of this right ensures that people have a right to determine how they should live their lives and more importantly how and when they wish to end their lives. However, there are problems with how this right is interpreted, especially when it is applied to advanced directives.

Advanced directives

Due to a fear among many people that there may come a stage in their lives when they will no longer be competent to make decisions regarding their health and the medical care they require, the idea of advanced directives began to evolve. These documents are meant to act as guides to families and the medical profession. They can request the termination, withdrawal or non-provision of health care. In most cases, they are intended to take effect in the event of the person who drew up the document becoming incompetent (i.e. unable to make rational decisions). There are a number of ways in which advanced directives can be instituted. They can be in the form of a *living will* which requests and directs that certain measures should, or more particularly, should not, be taken if someone becomes incompetent or ill in some way specified in the document (e.g. 'terminally' or 'irreversibly' ill). An alternative to a *living will* is an *enduring power of attorney*. This document appoints an agent to take decisions of specific types in specified situations in the event of one's incompetence through accident, disease or injury. There can also be a document containing both a *living will* and an *enduring power of attorney*.

Since 1976, most states in the United States have legislated to give legal effect to living wills, and all states have provided for enduring powers of attorney. In Australia, the state of Victoria enacted in 1988–9 a Medical Treatment Act sharing many, but not all, of the features common among the American statutes. In the United Kingdom, the Voluntary Euthanasia Society launched a 'Medical Treatment (Advanced Directives) Bill' in 1991 which was intended to enable people to give directions to their physicians regarding the withholding or withdrawal of life-sustaining treatment in the event of a terminal disease.[87]

A characteristic moral argument for giving compulsory moral and legal effect to advanced directives is offered in *The Living Will: Consent to Treatment at the End of Life*.[88] This report, known at the Kennedy Report, argues that a patient is entitled to refuse any form of treatment, even if death is the inevitable outcome. It takes the view that even if the patient is not suffering from a terminal illness from which they would otherwise die, starvation is not suicide. The patient must positively do something to themselves, such as the refusal of treatment or nourishment, before their conduct would be so regarded. Furthermore, even if the law were to regard the patient as committing suicide, the doctor's omission to continue artificial feeding or hydration would not be regarded as 'assistance'. This follows because the doctor must act to commit the offence and not merely omit to do something, and because the patient's refusal absolves the doctor of any duty in law to continue treatment.[89]

According to John Finnis the pervasive error of principle in the Kennedy Report is the refusal to consider the significance of intention. The primary question is not whether death is an 'inevitable outcome', but whether death is intended, that is whether the patient intends to die as a means of escaping suffering and/or of securing some advantage. If the patient does, his or her plan to refuse medical treatment or nourishment is suicidal, and the doctors' decisions accordingly to withhold treatment or nourishment are decisions to aid and abet. According to English law, a refusal which is motivated by suicidal intent is unlawful, even though suicide itself is not a criminal offence; that is why assistance, and agreements to assist, in suicide are serious criminal offences.[90]

Jim Stone in a detailed article 'Advanced Directives, Autonomy and Unintended Death', writes that living wills have two defects. First, most living wills fail to enable people to avoid unwanted medical intervention effectively. Second, most living wills have the potential danger of ending lives in ways people never intended, years before the person would naturally die. Policy issues surrounding advanced directives often seem pretty obvious and simple, when in fact they are extremely complicated and difficult. Partly as a consequence, living wills and other advanced directives tend to be badly directed, vague and confusing to lay people, lawyers and the medical professionals who implement them. People generally do not understand the implications of the advanced directives they sign, or, for that matter, create.[91]

THE PRACTICE OF EUTHANASIA IN THE NETHERLANDS

The Netherlands has been in the 'euthanasia headlines' for the last fourteen years. This is due to their current practice of facilitating requests for voluntary euthanasia. According to Dutch law, the intentional killing of a person at their 'express and serious' request is an offence contrary to Article 293 of the Dutch Penal Code, and assisting suicide is prohibited by the following Article. However, in 1981, in response to the growing demand and practice of euthanasia by the medical profession, the Rotterdam criminal court set out certain guidelines for euthanasia which, if followed, would be unlikely to render the doctor concerned liable for prosecution. Since then Dutch courts have held that doctors charged with either offence can successfully avail themselves of the defence of necessity if they have acted in accordance with 'responsible medical opinion' measured by the 'prevailing standards of medical ethics'.[92]

When, according to 'responsible medical opinion', is it considered appropriate for a doctor to carry out euthanasia? In 1984 the Royal Dutch Medical Association published a report setting out conditions in which 'euthanasia' (a word which is used in Holland to mean 'voluntary euthanasia') accorded with medical ethics. It specified five conditions:

1   The request must be made of the patient's free will, and not result from pressure by others.
2   The request must be 'well-considered', and not based on a misunderstanding of diagnosis or prognosis.
3   The request must be 'durable', and not arise from impulse or temporary depression.
4   The patient must be experiencing 'unacceptable suffering';

he must feel the suffering to be 'persistent, unbearable and hopeless'.

5   The doctor must consult with a colleague before performing euthanasia, and report it to the legal authorities afterwards as a non-natural death.[93]

Finally in 1993, the Dutch parliament ratified this practice in a law which stopped short of making euthanasia legal but declared that doctors would not be prosecuted if they followed the procedures and restrictions the law set out. Dr Admiraal, an advocate and practitioner of euthanasia, while pointing out that justifiable active euthanasia is practised in the Netherlands only with patients who are in the terminal phase of an incurable and usually malignant disease, examines why patients request this act.[94] He finds that it occurs usually when patients find that their sufferings have become unbearable. But what constitutes unbearable suffering? Normally it has two closely related causes: physical and psychological pain. The physical causes include:

1   Loss of strength which is sometimes so severe that the patient becomes totally incapable of any physical exertion.

2   Fatigue, even without physical effort, which is experienced as exhaustion.

3   Shortness of breath as a result of lung aberrations or tumours in the trachea or mouth cavity.

4   Nausea and vomiting resulting from a blockage of the oesophagus or gastrointestinal tract.

5   Incontinence, sleeplessness and pain.

6   'Cancer pain' which refers to real physical pain combined with fear, sorrow, depression and exhaustion. This kind of pain is an alarm signal indicating shortcomings in inter-human contact and misunderstandings of the patient's situation. This 'pain' can be treated with good terminal care based on warm human contact.

Physical pain can be adequately controlled in most cases with morphine-like analgesics and/or psycho-pharmaceuticals, which block sensitive or sympathetic nervous tissue without adversely affecting the normal psychological functions of the patient. Thus physical pain alone, according to Admiraal, does not medically justify euthanasia. Psychological pain results from the above-mentioned somatic problems. It also includes anxieties about pain and suffering, about spiritual and physical deformation, about becoming completely dependent and needing total nursing care, and about dying itself. It includes grief about the loss of family and possessions; sorrow when grief is bottled up and not understood by others; and bitter grief when the patient asks why this happens to them at this point in their lives. Grief can turn into rancour, revolt, aggression and depression. These factors combine to facilitate the total disintegration of humanness and cause unbearable suffering. Thus, according to Dr Admiraal, 'euthanasia in our hospitals is a dignified last act of assistance to the patient in his terminal phase'.[95]

However another influential physician, Dr Jan Hendrick van den Berg, suggested that doctors should not just assist consenting patients to die, but should also be obliged to take 'meaningless lives' without patient consent. Evidently 77% of the Dutch public, according to one poll, supported not just active killing by physicians of patients who are able to consent (voluntary euthanasia), but active killing by physicians of patients who are unable to consent and have slipped into a low quality of life (involuntary euthanasia). There is therefore a fear that once active euthanasia becomes legalised, it will be demanded for the incompetent as well.[96]

Even though 80% of Dutch people support the right to die, and the Dutch practice has been approved and warmly defended by the Royal Dutch Medical Association, foreign doctors and commentators, it has also been heavily criticised.[97] In an attempt to answer these criticisms, especially the criticism that theirs was a widespread breach of the guidelines, an investigation was instituted. In 1991 the Dutch Governmental Commission on Euthanasia, chaired by Attorney-General Remmelink, published its report.[98] This survey appears to demonstrate that doctors either practised euthanasia or intentionally intended to shorten the life of their patients in almost 20,000 cases. There also seemed to be evidence that in some cases doctors certified death by natural causes when they had in fact used euthanasia, thereby breaching the fifth guideline.[99] This led Dr Carlos Gomez to conclude that the Dutch attempts to control euthanasia and to provide for public accountability have failed and that attempts to protect vulnerable patients have proved 'halfhearted and ineffective at best'.[100] Instead of helping and protecting and being an advocate of the vulnerable, physicians are in danger of becoming a threat to the sick and dying patients. Dr John Keown also found that not only had the guidelines been widely ignored, but that killing, even without request, was now officially approved of. Evidence for this can be found in recent publications of the Royal Dutch Medical Association which approved, in certain circumstances, the killing of handicapped neonates and patients in comas, and, most recently, those with severe dementia.[101]

One would have expected that the publication of the Remmelink Report, especially the non-reporting of cases of euthanasia, would have had a detrimental impact on Dutch society, especially on patient-doctor relations. But according to Chris Ciesielski-Carlucci and Gerrit Kimsma, there has been no noticeable change in Dutch society's view of the medical profession. However they point out that in order for the physician to act in a way that is in concert with professional codes, societal norms and legal requirements, all cases of euthanasia should be reported. Lack of reporting complicates both the experience and process of euthanasia, whereas reporting fosters an environment of trust which greatly reduces the occurrence of these complications. They go on to argue that 'a policy of openness, which can only occur through the reporting of euthanasia is beneficial to families, beneficial to physicians and society, and after all, is consistent with the Dutch philosophy in handling controversial issues'.[102]

The criteria for euthanasia appear to have been extended by another case which occurred in 1994. In this case Dr Chabot, a Dutch psychiatrist, administered a lethal dose to a 50-year-old woman who appeared to be 'suffering unacceptably' without any prospect of relief. This woman, who was estranged from her husband, had been through the trauma of the suicide of both her sons and could not envisage a life without them. She had already attempted suicide and stated that she wanted to die. Dr Chabot found no evidence of severe psychosis or personality disorder. He nevertheless believed that with or without his help her wish to die was genuine. He sought further medical advice and arrived at the conclusion that her determination to die was well considered and consistent. He then assisted her to die by administering a yoghurt-type dessert spiked with a lethal dose.

Dr Chabot was charged under the Dutch Penal Code, but both the local court and the appeal court dismissed charges against him. But the Ministry of Justice chose to take a test case to the Supreme Court. At the heart of the case lay the concern that Dr Chabot's patient was not physically, terminally ill. Neither was it felt possible to judge if someone is 'suffering unacceptably' when the source of the suffering is mental rather than physical. However, prior to the Supreme Court judgment the Royal Dutch Medical Association published guidelines on assisted suicide for psychiatric patients in November 1993. These guidelines accepted that there may be cases where it is merciful to assist by suicide or voluntary euthanasia patients who have serious psychiatric problems if there is no prospect of improvement. In the Dr Chabot case, the Supreme Court came to the unusual but pragmatic conclusion that Dr Chabot was guilty but would not be punished. His failure to insist that a second doctor should have examined his patient meant the court refused to accept that he had acted in an emergency, which was his particular line of defence. But, it added, there were special reasons why it would not punish Dr Chabot. These related to the previous judgment of the appeal court, which accepted that Dr Chabot had acted reliably in consulting with colleagues and that he had attempted to persuade his patient to reject suicide.

This case not only raises new ethical issues but also sets a new euthanasia precedent. Now it appears that a patient need not be in a 'terminal phase' of life, or intolerable suffering from physical and psychological pain for euthanasia to be considered. This expansion of the criteria governing euthanasia in the

Netherlands has been welcomed by the Dutch Society for Voluntary Euthanasia and the Royal Dutch Medical Association.[103]

CHRISTIAN TRADITION REGARDING EUTHANASIA

The Christian churches make a substantial case against any form of euthanasia, appealing to both religious and secular principles. While there are significant common arguments, their different approaches demonstrate the richness of the Christian tradition. Yet it should also be noted that divergent views are expressed by theologians who attempt to move the debate into the relational and contextual spheres of life. This is particularly evident when the distinction between ordinary and extraordinary means are discussed and the problems of hydration and nutrition are addressed.

Roman Catholic Church

The teaching authority of the Roman Catholic Church demonstrates a continual opposition to euthanasia. This teaching is founded on the nature of human existence as a gift from God which is protected by God's commands. Thus when the Second Vatican Council taught on this issue it was recalling a constant and firm Christian teaching on the reverence due to human life. In *Gaudium et spes* the Council Fathers declared that whatever is opposed to life itself 'such as any type of murder, genocide, abortion, euthanasia and wilful suicide . . . all these and the like are criminal; they poison civilisation, and they debase the perpetrators more than the victims and militate against the honour of the creator'.[104]

The Council did not elaborate on what it understood euthanasia to be. Rather it referred back to the two previous explanations given by Pope Pius XII in 1957. In the first of these, the Pope considered the use of pain-relieving drugs and explained how they need not amount to euthanasia even if the use of the drugs, for the sake of relieving pain, might shorten the life of a dying person. But he made it quite clear that the use of drugs with the direct intention of procuring or hastening death was immoral.[105] In the second address, Pius XII considered the use of techniques of artificial respiration on deeply unconscious patients who, if not already dead, would certainly die a few minutes after any cessation of the techniques. His argument emphasised the rights and duties of the patient, the doctor and the patient's family. He began by stating that natural reason and Christian morals affirms that all persons and those entrusted with their care had the right and duty, in cases of serious illness, to make use of whatever treatment was necessary for the preservation of life. But this duty normally obliges one only to the use of ordinary means, according to the circumstances of persons, places, epochs and culture; that is, of means that do not impose any extraordinary burden on the person or on someone else. Since extraordinary forms of treatment go beyond the ordinary means which one is bound to have recourse to, it cannot be maintained that there is any obligation to use them or, consequently, to authorise one's doctor to use them. The rights and duties of the patient's family are based on the presumed will of the unconscious patient if he or she is elderly or unable to make decisions. As to the family's own independent duty, the only obligation in normal circumstances is to employ ordinary means. Consequently, if it were to appear that any attempted resuscitation constituted a burden on the family such as one could not in conscience impose on them, they can legitimately insist that the doctor cease his or her attempts, and the doctor can legitimately comply. In cases like this, Pius insists that there is no direct disposal of the life of the patient, no euthanasia.[106]

The teaching of Pius XII provides a clear indication of what the Second Vatican Council had in mind when it condemned euthanasia. Since the Council, the magisterium has given a further expression of its teaching and the theological basis upon which it is founded. *The Declaration on Euthanasia* issued by the Congregation for the Doctrine of the Faith on 5 May 1980 provides a fuller treatment of the subject. It begins by stating that euthanasia is an 'action or omission which of itself or by intention causes death, in order that all suffering may in this way be eliminated. Euthanasia's terms of reference, therefore, are to be found in the intention of the will and the methods used.'[107] It goes on to point out that phrases such as 'mercy killing', 'rational suicide', 'physician-assisted suicide' and the like should not be allowed to obscure the fact that euthanasia is the killing of an innocent human being and, as such, is morally wrong and should not be condoned by any civilised society. The *Declaration*'s opposition to euthanasia is based on two arguments. First, that 'human life is the basis of all goods, and is the necessary source and condition of every human activity and of society'. Since most people regard life as something sacred no one has the right to dispose of it at will. The second argument concerns those who have faith. 'Believers', it says, 'see in life something greater, namely a gift from God's love, which they are called upon to preserve and make fruitful.'[108] This being so, the teaching concludes, euthanasia 'is a question of the violation of the divine law, an offence against the dignity of the human person, a crime against life, and an attack on humanity'.[109]

In its rejection of suicide and euthanasia, it also addressed the extent to which there is an obligation to sustain life. The *Declaration* states that everyone has the duty to care for his or her own health or to seek such care from others. Those whose task it is to care for the sick must do so conscientiously and administer the remedies that seem necessary or useful. It ends this section with a question about whether it is necessary in all circumstances to have recourse to all possible remedies?[110] The complexities involved in responding to this question will be fully explored in the sections on 'ordinary' and 'extraordinary means' and 'nutrition and hydration'.

The *Catechism* elaborates on the points already raised when it states that whatever its motives and means, direct euthanasia consists in putting an end to the lives of handicapped, sick or dying persons: it is morally unacceptable. It then goes on to look at three areas of controversy. The first concerns intentional omission of treatment. In this instance it teaches that 'an act or omission which, of itself or by intention, causes death in order to eliminate suffering constitutes a murder gravely contrary to the dignity of the human person and of the respect due to the living God, his Creator'. The second deals with medical procedures.

Once again it refers back to Pius XII and states that 'discontinuing medical procedures that are burdensome, dangerous, extraordinary, or disproportionate to the expected outcome can be legitimate; it is the refusal of "over-zealous" treatment'. In these cases the physician does not intend to cause death, rather it is an acceptance of death and of the inability to impede it. Decisions of this sort should be made by the patient if they are competent or by those legally entitled to act for them. However it goes on to insist that 'even if death is thought imminent, the ordinary care owed to a sick person cannot be legitimately interrupted'. Painkillers to alleviate the sufferings of the dying, even at the risk of shortening their lives, can be used. But there should not be the intention in using them to either hasten death or cause death; rather their use and effects although foreseen should be tolerated as an inevitable way of alleviating suffering.[111]

In his recent encyclical *Evangelium Vitae* John Paul II writes that euthanasia in the strict sense must be understood to be an action or omission which of itself and by intention causes death, with the purpose of eliminating all suffering. 'Euthanasia's terms of reference, therefore, are to be found in the intention of the will and the methods used.'[112] He goes on to 'confirm that euthanasia is a grave violation of the law of God, since it is the deliberate and morally unacceptable killing of a human person. This doctrine is based upon the natural law and upon the written word of God, is transmitted by the Church's Tradition and taught by the ordinary and universal Magisterium.' Depending on the circumstances, this practice involves the malice proper to suicide or murder.[113]

However, unlike the encyclical's treatment of abortion its teaching on euthanasia is more practical and more in tune with clinical realities. This is demonstrated by the distinctions the Pope draws. He argues that euthanasia must be distinguished from the decision to forgo so-called 'aggressive medical treatment', in other words, medical procedures which no longer correspond to the real situation of the patient, either because they are by now disproportionate to any expected results or because they impose an excessive burden on the patient and his or her family. In such situations, when death is clearly imminent and inevitable, one can in conscience 'refuse forms of treatment that would only secure a precarious and burdensome prolongation of life, so long as the normal care due to the sick person in similar cases is not interrupted'. To forgo extraordinary or disproportionate means is not the equivalent of suicide or euthanasia; it rather expresses acceptance of the human condition in the face of death.

In referring to modern methods of palliative care which seek to make suffering more bearable in the final stages of illness and to ensure that the patient is supported and accompanied in his or her ordeal, the Pope raises the question of the licitness of using various types of painkillers and sedatives for relieving the patient's pain when this involves the risk of shortening life. John Paul II follows the teaching of Pope Pius XII by affirming that it is licit to relieve pain by narcotics, even when the result is decreased consciousness and a shortening of life, 'if no other means exist, and if, in the given circumstances, this does not prevent the carrying out of other religious and moral duties'. In such a case death is not willed or sought, there is simply a desire to ease pain effectively by using the analgesics which medicine provides.[114]

Theological development

The following principles underline the theological arguments against suicide and euthanasia: they are considered as offences against the exclusive right of disposition by God the Creator over the life and death of a human being; they also offend against the good of society and contradict self-love.

In traditional moral theology, the exclusive right of disposition by God over creation is the most important and most conclusive argument. Pope John Paul II often refers to this principle when he teaches that human life is a unique value in the whole of creation. God, in fact, created everything for people. The person is 'the only creature that God wanted for its own sake'.[115] Therefore only God can 'dispose' of this extraordinary gift of life. The human being only possesses life as a gift. The Pope goes on to point out that this giftedness is defended in the Ten Commandments which teach 'You shall not kill' (Ex. 20:13). The Scriptures immediately afterwards add a clarification stating 'Do not slay the innocent and righteous, for I will not acquit the wicked' (Ex. 23:7). This teaching is also emulated by Christ when he confirms this commandment as a condition to 'enter life' (Mt. 19:18). Significantly, Christ follows it with the commandment that sums up every aspect of the moral law—the commandment of love (Mt. 19:19).[116]

Theology argues that God's creation and sustaining of creation is a gift because it is utterly free and unconstrained. For human beings not only is this life a great gift but it is also accompanied by responsibilities. Humanity honours, serves and loves God by respecting, fostering and loving the goods he has created and put in our charge. The gifts of creation, particularly the goods of human existence, are to be developed, fostered and actively protected against whatever threatens them. That is why when medical care is necessary and available, people are morally obliged to have recourse to it, up to the point where it becomes futile, or where it would itself involve burdens that the patient need not feel obliged to undergo.[117]

In recent years, however, the absolute conclusive force of this argument has increasingly been undermined. The challenge is not based on the understanding of God as the ultimate owner of the human body and life, but rather on a new understanding of the human person's co-creative role with God in life. Human life demonstrates that we can and do dispose of parts of our bodies in amputations, and that at times we actually sacrifice human life in war. This means that the human person cannot arbitrarily dispose of these things, rather actions must be in conformity with the task given them by God within the framework of the unfolding divine plan for creation and the realisation of his kingdom of love and justice. This has led some authors[118] to conclude that active, direct euthanasia can be justified in certain circumstances. These circumstances would include the preservation of a person's freedom and dignity when threatened by an excruciating illness, or out of compassion and fraternal love for the person suffering. Other theologians do not go as far as this but concede that for borderline cases an entirely straight ethical solution cannot always be found.[119] However, a solution must be located within the circumstances and conditions in which patients find themselves. Thus it might be possible, within strict conditions and circumstances, to assist someone to die. Traditional theology answers this challenge by arguing that human stewardship of life does not include the choice to terminate the stewardship itself. The conditions of stewardship, then, are provided by God's commandments or mandates. Men and women can come to a knowledge of these commandments by conscientious exercise of natural reason, even without the benefit of God's self-disclosure to Israel and through Jesus. In that self-disclosure there is revealed a commandment which, as explained through Scripture and the tradition of the Church, forbids human beings to intend the termination of life. It is argued that it has always been the Christian belief that the expression of God's will holds good in all circumstances and conditions of life.[120]

Other theologians such as McCormick,[121] Holderegger,[122] Rotter,[123] who do not refer to the property rights of God over the human person reject active euthanasia from the principle of the common good and self-love.

The first argument, based on the principle of the common good, emphasises the danger of escalation. It is feared that legalisation of voluntary euthanasia would create a precedent to extend the practice to handicapped and sick individuals also, who do not suffer so much themselves, but rather are a burden to society. Whether or not there is such a danger depends on the basic approach of those who are in favour of euthanasia. Kevin Kelly points out that although many supporters of voluntary euthanasia base their case on respect for the freedom of the individual human being, it may well be that their understanding of who qualifies for the category of 'human being' depends on the quality of human life present. If this were so, it would be logical for them to regard the state as an institution whose duty it was to safeguard and promote the common good of 'good quality human beings' and dispose of those who do not meet the agreed criteria.[124]

The second argument centres on the fundamental value of trust between the physician and patient which could seriously suffer and possibly perish, if physicians could practise mercy killing. Furthermore, there could be a detrimental effect upon medical progress if euthanasia were regarded as an acceptable solution to medical problems. Yet it can be counter-argued that such a loss of trust will only come about if euthanasia is practised against the will of a patient who is in principle competent. A similar situation already exists when life-prolonging measures are discontinued, a step admitted by all ethicists for adequate reasons. However, there is always the danger that life-prolonging measures could be discontinued too early in order to gain organs for transplant. In spite of this danger, there has not been a loss of trust in the medical profession. This is due to the fact that appropriate norms have been instituted which prevent possible abuses. The evidence from the Netherlands, at this stage of the practice, also appears to demonstrate that there has not been any fundamental breakdown in the trust between physicians and patients.

The third argument concentrates on the free consent of the patient. The question raised is: How can consent be discerned and is it actually free? Some physicians point out that the wish of the sick person for euthanasia is often only a hidden plea for more help and more personal concern and care, or the result of a temporary depression or a momentary disturbance caused by heavy medication. This wish, they argue, disappears when better help and personal care are provided.[125] Finally, the wish could also be the result of an imagined or real social pressure. An old person, for instance, who is suffering from an incurable terminal disease might feel a kind of moral obligation to request euthanasia in order to relieve the burden imposed on relatives. Certain precautions are possible to guard against such dangers, such as the offering of better care; an adequate waiting period before euthanasia is initiated, and consultation between the physician in charge with another physician. Nevertheless the possibility of social pressure is a serious danger. If free consent is seen as a basic prerequisite for euthanasia, what about those patients who are unable to consent, such as minors and newborns, who suffer from severe pains of an illness or of a defect? Can consent in such cases be given by the parents or another proxy? This would be euthanasia without free consent of the patient, although it is not necessarily against the will of the patient. A step in this direction could initiate social euthanasia. The fear is that once it is embarked upon it will be impossible to control.

The fourth argument from the common good is that euthanasia will have a harmful effect upon society. As long as human dignity is not based simply on usefulness to society, people such as the mentally ill, the severely handicapped, the very young and the incurably sick must be treated with respect and their lives safeguarded. An acceptance even of voluntary euthanasia 'would seem to involve a weakening of this basic position'.[126]

Professor Holderegger believes that euthanasia should be excluded on the grounds of self-love. He judges that 'the disposal of oneself seems justified as a gift and sacrifice for the life of another, while the direct causation of death because of a situation of privation is not justified'.[127] The reason for the prohibition lies in the person's vocation to realise their possibilities and to bring them to genuine fullness. In normal circumstances this reason does not raise major problems, but when considered in the context of physical and psychological suffering it needs to be questioned. What is at issue here is the meaning of suffering.

If it is true in an absolute way, as Holderegger suggests, that every agony of the dying has to be considered as a first phase of human maturing enveloped by God's affirmation which a person is not allowed to shorten, then this would exclude indirect abbreviation of life by narcotics and the passive omission of life-prolonging measures in order to alleviate a person's suffering. And yet these measures are generally considered morally lawful. From a merely humanistic point of view, self-love seems to be a weighty argument for the shortening of suffering, where no hope of recovery exists. Although life is the most fundamental, temporal good of a person, it is not the highest good at all. In principle the liberation from suffering is a good, because it is the object of all the works of mercy. Yet is the liberation from grave, terminal suffering a good which justifies a termination of life by euthanasia? Here opinions diverge.[128] According to Christian teaching, 'suffering, especially suffering during the last moments of life, has a special place in God's saving plan; it is in fact a sharing in Christ's passion and a union with the redeeming sacrifice which he offered in obedience to the Father's will'.[129]

But there are instances of 'total pain',[130] where even under the most favourable conditions of good caring and intensive personal care (conditions which often are wanting) the sufferings cannot be mastered and the wish for assistance to die does not fall silent. Unbearable suffering or 'total pain', as pointed out by Dr Admiraal, has normally two closely related causes: physical and psychological pain. Physical pain can be adequately controlled in most cases with drugs. Psychological pain which can result from physical pain includes, for many patients, anxieties about pain and suffering, about spiritual and physical deformity, about becoming completely dependent and needing total nursing care, and about dying itself. It includes grief about loss of family and grief about why this is happening to them. When physical pain and psychological pain combine they facilitate the total disintegration of humanness and cause unbearable suffering.[131] Can unbearable suffering, both physical and mental, be considered as redemptive in these circumstances?

What should be apparent from our discussion is that some authors emphasise the value of life above all else. However, there is always the danger that this might be absolutised in a somewhat rigid manner. This would be contrary to the Christian tradition which teaches that life is a fundamental value but not an absolute one. Very little consideration is given by some authors to persons and relationships. Professor Lisa Sowle Cahill addresses this particular issue when she writes that the Christian tradition envisions life as a fundamental value but not an absolute one. This is why causing death can be a form of respect for life, and particularly for the total dignity and welfare of persons, which include spiritual as well as physical aspects. This same tradition has limited causation to indirect means although that limit is the subject of ongoing discussion among those who see relief of suffering as a duty of love which can in exceptional cases outweigh the stringent duty not to destroy life directly.[132]

If emphasis is placed on relational values it might be possible to envisage a situation in which the interests of a particular patient might be best served by assisting that person to die. A greater emphasis on relationships between doctors and patients may also help to overcome the danger of abuse which is referred to so often when discussing euthanasia. It should be possible to contemplate the possibility that, in meeting the demands of the doctor-patient relationship by helping the patient to die, a physician may be expressing something entirely positive.

Criticism is aimed at this relational approach because it highlights the danger of confining itself to individual ethics which are based on primarily subjective grounds. Euthanasia is, however, fundamentally a problem of social ethics[133] and concerns all basic human relationships, not just the interpersonal doctor-patient one. At an individual level it may be possible to argue in favour of it, but the possible effect on social life, such as undermining the ethos of the caring profession, the implications for the family and society, seem to militate against legislating in favour of it.

The Church of England

In 1936 and 1969 two voluntary euthanasia bills were presented to the British Parliament. In response to the growing pressure to legalise voluntary euthanasia the Church of England's Board for Social Responsibility set up a working party to investigate voluntary euthanasia. The fruits of this working party were published in 1975. This document, *On Dying Well*, represents a model of how the question of the care for the dying should be addressed.[134]

The report begins by registering a 'strong dissent from the use of the expression "right to die".' It takes exception to its use in the euthanasia debate because it 'suffers from a dangerous ambiguity'. It can mean that a person has the right to determine whether he or she should live or die, which implies that a person can claim assistance from the medical profession in bringing about their death. It can also mean that an individual can consent to the doctor ending their life, where pain cannot be controlled. Finally, it can mean that patients *in extremis* should not be subjected to troublesome treatments which cannot restore them to health, and doctors may use drugs to control pain even at the risk of shortening life.[135]

The report goes on to admit that there are extreme situations outside the medical field, such as soldiers fatally trapped in a blazing gun-turret, or wounded individuals who face certain death by torture, where it is impossible to say that those who have killed them to prevent pain have acted wrongfully. However, the authors are reluctant to admit such exceptions exist in medicine. They point out that even if there were, it would be impossible to specify them precisely enough to prevent continuous and abusive expansion. This point of view was supported by the then Bishop of Durham, the Right Reverend J. S. Habgood, who cautioned that the consequences of legislation permitting euthanasia would, in the long run, be 'incalculable', not least because of the likely failure of any safeguards to prevent abuse.[136] For this reason, the report argues, 'a professional ethics cannot be built on altogether exceptional circumstances, even if in some such exceptional cases a man who contravenes it might rightly be held not to be morally culpable'.[137]

The report goes on to insist that there is a difference between killing and relieving the pain of the dying, whether by withholding life support or by administering pain relievers that may hasten death. In this, they are echoing Pius XII and the tradition that preceded and followed him. There is a clear distinction 'to be drawn between rendering someone unconscious at the risk of killing him and killing him to render him unconscious'. Killing involves a 'definite and in its implications momentous change of policy'. The authors agree that those who do not have to make decisions 'regard such discrimination as unnecessarily fine, but its importance tends to be intuitively evident to those upon whom the burden of decisions rests'. Thus it would seem that the report appeals to intuitive experience to establish the moral significance between killing and allowing to die.

Finally, the report faces the euthanasist plea for compassion. The authors admit that the plea is a deeply human and a highly moral one and must not fall on deaf ears. But they then insist that the value of human life does not consist simply of a scale of pleasure and pain. Rather, the value of human life consists in a variety of virtues and graces as well as in pleasure. Therefore, what a person consists of is not only what he or she does, but also how he or she endures. 'A fully human life is inescapably vulnerable, as every lover knows, and even suffering may by grace be woven into the texture of a large humanity.' The authors point out that this does not mean that suffering is in itself good, or that it necessarily ennobles. But that 'suffering as exposure to what is beyond one's voluntary control, suffering as undergoing, even as diminishment, is part of the pattern of becoming human. Even dying need not be simply the ebbing away of life; it may be integrated into life and so made instrumental to a fuller life in God.'[138] This understanding of suffering provides the context for the use of technology in care. The context is one that refuses to absolutise any one consideration and thereby represents a more fully human response to the condition of the dying person.

The authors of the report go on to emphasise that human beings live in interdependence. They point out that in life

there is a movement of giving and receiving. At the beginning and at the end of life receiving predominates over and even excludes giving. But the value of human life does not depend only on its capacity to give. Love, *agape*, is the equal and unalterable regard for the value of other human beings independent of their particular characteristics. It extends especially to the helpless and hopeless, to those who have no value in their own eyes and seemingly none in the eyes of society. Such neighbour-love is costly and sacrificial. It is easily destroyed. In the giver it demands unlimited caring, in the recipient absolute trust. The question must be asked whether the practice of voluntary euthanasia is consistent with the fostering of such caring and trust.[139]

The authors of the report *On Dying Well* realised that their arguments would not foreclose the moral debate but 'they are sufficient . . . to show that there are strong grounds from the Christian point of view for hesitating long before admitting any exception to the principle forbidding killing human beings'.[140]

In 1992 the House of Bishops recognised that there was a need for further guidance concerning the theological, ethical and social implications of euthanasia. Its statement was meant to complement the work already done by the Board for Social Responsibility in the light of the changes that had taken place since the 1975 report *On Dying Well*. The bishops therefore wished to reaffirm the principles underlying the earlier report, which they believed must remain the foundation of public policy. Yet they recognised that within the complexity of the matters which have to be considered in individual cases, decisions must always remain a matter of moral judgment. They argued that because human life is a gift from God to be preserved and nourished, the deliberate taking of human life is prohibited except in self-defence or the legitimate defence of others. When addressing the distinction between deliberate killing and the administration of painkilling drugs or withdrawal of treatment that may have the effect of shortening life, the bishops affirmed that the sanctity of life must remain the guiding principle. This would ensure the proper self-understanding of the medical profession as protectors of life and maintain the necessary public confidence in the medical profession. In referring to the medical possibility of keeping people alive in circumstances where death might otherwise have brought relief from intolerable suffering, they point out that doctors do not have an overriding obligation to prolong life by all available means. Crucial decisions in such circumstances should be made collaboratively and should involve more than one medically qualified person.

They go on to argue that it is a Christian imperative and a duty of the state to protect the interests of the most vulnerable, particularly those who may feel themselves to be burdensome to others or unwanted, and who thus might be under pressure to seek the hastening of their own deaths. Human autonomy is limited, they argue, and thus what human beings may do to themselves or require others to do for them should be guided by specifically religious considerations such as the God-given character of human life and the social consequences of individual actions on other people, whether directly or indirectly through the gradual shift of social perceptions and expectations. The House of Bishops, therefore, urged great caution before any attempt is made to change public policy. In commending the Hospice movement, they pointed out that given appropriate care and the use of modern techniques developed within the movement, the vast majority of the dying can do so with dignity and without pain.[141]

The Church of Scotland

The Church of Scotland affirms that people owe their physical and spiritual existence to God alone and that God must remain in control over life. Ultimate authority in matters of life and death rests solely with God from whom that life derives. It follows then that a person's life is not his or her property; it is a loan. As such it must be held in trust. In the broadest sense, it is meant for the service of God.[142]

The primary and fundamental principle is that of the sanctity of human life. This is a principle long recognised in all societies based on the Judeo-Christian ethic, in most, if not all civilised societies, and in most other religious systems, including Islam and Hinduism. It is enshrined in Article 2 of the *European*

Convention for the Protection of Human Rights and Fundamental Freedoms (1953), and in Article 6 of the *International Covenant of Civil and Political Rights* (1966). Fundamental though it is, however, this is not an absolute principle in law. There are recognised exceptions (for example, it may be lawful to take the life of another in self-defence) but, where the principle is applicable, the law takes the view that causing the death of another with intent to do so is murder.[143] Thus the Board for Social Responsibility of the Church of Scotland argues that legalising euthanasia will not produce a solution to the needs of the individual sufferer nor would it address the health-care challenges of contemporary society. Rather it is the expression of an attitude to life which belittles the sovereignty of God, diminishes the importance of sustaining relationships, and inhibits the pursuit of life-affirming answers for people in need and in distress. Christians, they argue, must be active in promoting positive alternatives derived from biblical truth in order that the momentum toward intentional killing may be curbed. The Board goes on to affirm that the Church of Scotland has an obligation before God to assert God's affirmation of life, to exercise Christian compassion towards the sufferer, the disabled and the dying and to encourage the relief of symptoms and improvement in the quality of life for such people. The Board therefore decided that it could not support euthanasia as a means to any of these ends, and rejected the introduction of death as a treatment option in any clinical situation.[144]

The Methodist Church

The Methodist Church begins its analysis of euthanasia with a scriptural approach which holds that the life of a person bears the stamp of the God who 'made man in his own image' (Gen. 1:27). Therefore a person is meant to have fellowship with God and this relationship is an essential aspect of his or her life. It is, in fact, the possibility of an utterly unbreakable fellowship with God that gives a person's life its eternal dimension. Death is an event in that life, marking a transition rather than a terminus. For a Christian in fellowship with God, there is no 'terminal condition'. Death is part of life.

The Christian, therefore, approaches the euthanasia debate with many biblical strands: the dignity of the person deriving from unbroken fellowship with God; the eternal dimension of life which sets death in perspective; the call to use all God's gifts responsibly including the powers humans have over the lives of others; and above all the need to find in every situation the way of compassion. Some steps which can be taken immediately are obvious. Compassion must be shown through a much more energetic approach to problems of terminal care. Responsibility must be shouldered in the light of a new consideration of the appropriateness of certain forms of medical intervention. Despite its high cost in terms of time, money and pastoral care, this compassion and responsibility must be exercised by the medical services, the churches and society as a whole. The need is not so much to change the law as to alter the attitude of society towards death. This is an event which must be talked about and prepared for physically, mentally and spiritually. The families of the dying must be supported not only by the statutory services but also by the community. Pre-death loneliness must be relieved and those who are in the latter days of life must feel that they are still part of the family of God. The use of drugs and the increasing skills of medicine must be coupled with an understanding of the needs of the whole person. The spirit of the person also requires care and the Christian must be ready to respond to this need in his or her personal ministry. They point out that the artificial precipitation of death is likely to remain abhorrent to many people and this underpins their theological perspective on death which considers euthanasia to be both inappropriate and irrelevant.[145]

In 1993, in an act of ecumenical solidarity, the Church of England's House of Bishops, the Catholic Bishops' Conference of England and Wales and the leaders of the Free Churches in England made a public joint submission to the House of Lords Select Committee on Medical Ethics. In this submission they stated that they believed that God himself has given to humankind the gift of life. As such, it is to be revered and cherished. Christian beliefs about the special nature and value of human life lie at the root of the Western Christian humanist tradition, which remains greatly influential in shaping the values held by many in society. These beliefs are also shared in whole or in part by other faith communities. All human beings are to be valued, irrespective of age, sex, race, religion, social status or their potential for achievement. Those who become vulnerable through illness or disability deserve special care and protection. Adherence to this principle provides a fundamental test as to what constitutes a civilised society. The whole of humankind is the recipient of God's gift of life. It is to be received with gratitude and used responsibly. Human beings each have their own distinct identities but these are formed by and take their place within complex networks of relationships. All decisions about individual lives bear upon others with whom we live in community. For this reason, the law relating to euthanasia is not simply concerned either with private morality or with a utilitarian approach to life. On this issue there can be no moral pluralism. A positive choice has to be made by society in favour of protecting the interests of its vulnerable members even if this means limiting the freedom of others to determine their end.[146]

They concluded by saying that 'deliberately to kill a dying person would be to reject them'.[147] Because human life is a gift from God to be preserved and cherished, the deliberate taking of human life is prohibited except in self-defence or the legitimate defence of others. Therefore, all churches are resolutely opposed to legalising euthanasia even though it may be put forward as a means of relieving suffering, shortening the anguish of families or friends, or saving scarce resources.[148]

What the Christian churches argue for is the development of a society in which the true meaning of life and death can be understood. A caring community in which the need for euthanasia becomes irrelevant is a significant characteristic of such a society. Nobody would disagree with these aims, but the reality of our world still remains. People actually suffer and die without adequate medical and social care. Are the Christian churches ignoring this reality and the very real anguish that prolonged pain and suffering cause the afflicted person and those who have to co-endure this pain as they care for the sufferer?

CLARIFICATION OF CERTAIN POLEMICAL ISSUES

In our examination of the differing attitudes towards euthanasia certain disputed issues have emerged. These include the distinction between passive and active euthanasia; ordinary versus extraordinary means of medical treatment, and hydration and nutrition of people in a persistent vegetative state. A more detailed examination of these problematic issues might assist us in arriving at more fully informed moral decisions.

The distinction between active and passive euthanasia—killing or allowing to die

As has already been pointed out, the various church statements make a distinction between deliberate killing and the shortening of life through the administration of pain-killing drugs. Related to this is a fundamental ethical distinction between that which is intended, and that which is foreseen but unintended. For example, the administration of morphine is intended to relieve pain. The consequent shortening of life is foreseen but unintended. If safer drugs were available, they would be used: pain would be controlled and life would not be shortened.

There are many doctors who believe that passive euthanasia, either the withholding or withdrawal of treatment, is morally and legally preferable to active and deliberate intervention to cause the death of a patient. The *Declaration on Euthanasia* expands this belief by proposing that the treatment for a dying patient should be 'proportionate' to the therapeutic effect to be expected, and should not be disproportionately painful, intrusive, risky or costly, in the circumstances. Treatment may therefore be withheld or withdrawn. This is an area requiring fine judgment. Such decisions should be made collaboratively and by more than one medically qualified person. They should be guided by the principle that a pattern of care should never be adopted with the intention, purpose or aim of terminating the life or bringing about the death of a patient. Death, if it ensues, will have resulted from the underlying condition which required medical intervention.

The *Declaration* gives four concrete applications of this position.

1 If other remedies are not available, those as yet insufficiently tried may be used, with the consent of the patient, even though they may involve danger. Besides using them with the hope of being cured, the latter can accept them also with the hope of benefiting humanity.

2 It is also lawful to discontinue the use of such means when they are found not to justify the hope that was placed in them. In reaching this decision, account should be taken of the reasonable wishes of the patient, of the members of the family and of the skilled opinion of doctors. The latter should come to a proper judgment having taken into account the possible expenditure and effort required. The effect of treatment should be proportionately weighed against the suffering and inconvenience caused and the hoped-for possible advantage.

3 It is also permissible to make do with the normal means that medicine can offer. Therefore one cannot impose on anyone the obligation to have recourse to a technique which is already in use but which carries a risk or is burdensome. Such a refusal is not the equivalent of suicide; on the contrary, it should be considered as an acceptance of the human condition, or a wish to avoid the application of a medical procedure disproportionate to the results that can be expected, or a desire not to impose excessive expense on the family or the community.

4 Finally the *Declaration* points out that when death is imminent, and cannot be prevented by the remedies being used, the fact that treatments which involve only a precarious and painful prolonging of life can be conscientiously given up, does not mean that ordinary care which is available and given to patients in similar cases, may be interrupted. Where care for the dying person is thus

limited, doctors should not reproach themselves as though they had refused to help the person in danger of their life.[149] Albert Moraczewski accepts the relevance of the distinction.[150] In active euthanasia doctors are the cause of the death of their patients. 'Without intervention, death would not have ensued or ensued so quickly.' Contrarily, where artificial life-supports are removed, 'the individual was dying because of some existing pathology or injury'. The crucial point for Moraczewski is that active euthanasia 'brings about the patient's death'. It is the state of mind and intention that sets out actively to terminate life which is different from the person who sees that continued efforts to keep someone alive are to no avail.

Various philosophers and theologians challenge this distinction. Charles Curran argues that people have control over the dying process, because they can shorten the time of dying by not using or discontinuing even readily-available means of prolonging life. He asks is there really 'that great difference between this and positive interference to shorten the dying process?'[151] Paul Ramsey is more tentative, but suggests a time may come when the difference between commission (active) and omission (passive) disappears.[152] Richard McCormick agrees with Ramsey on the grounds that when (positive) care is no longer possible 'the difference between omission and commission would seem to lose moral meaning'.[153] However, neither Ramsey nor McCormick seem prepared to follow this view in practice, admitting, it seems, the practical impossibility of being certain that the point they postulate has actually been reached. Joseph Fletcher is far more strident in his argumentation stating that 'acts of deliberate omission are morally no different from acts of commission'.[154] Letting die by either the withholding or withdrawal of treatment can and does lead to needless cruelty and is a grotesque perversion of moral reasoning.[155]

James Rachels raises a number of arguments against the distinction.[156] Letting someone die may take a longer period of time, so the patient may suffer more than if direct action was taken. Thus, once the initial decision not to prolong life is made, active euthanasia is preferable. 'To say otherwise is to endorse the option that leads to more suffering rather than less and is contrary to the humanitarian impulse that prompts the decision not to prolong life in the first place.'

The belief that in active euthanasia the doctor does something, whereas in allowing someone to die the doctor merely ceases treatment, is challenged. Rachels argues that by allowing someone to die the doctor truly does something. He concludes by saying that the reason why it is considered bad to be the cause of someone's death is that death is regarded as a great evil. However, if it has been decided that euthanasia, even passive euthanasia, is desirable in a given case, it has also been decided that in this instance death is no greater an evil than the patient's continued existence. And if that is true, the real reason for not wanting to be the cause of someone's death simply does not apply.[157]

Peter Singer,[158] while agreeing with both Fletcher and Rachels, goes on to point out that when we get down to cases that embody a distinction between killing and letting die, then 'without any other irrelevant considerations to influence our judgment, it becomes implausible to say that there is a great moral difference between the act and the omission'. He offers several reasons for this conclusion. First, in either case 'we must take responsibility for what we do . . . a decision not to do something is as much a decision as one to do something'. Second, 'most people agree that this intuitive feeling [that it is worse to kill than to let die] is unreliable'. Finally, he argues that 'avoidance of pointless suffering must take precedence over a rigid adherence to a prohibition on killing'.

Due to the confusion and ambiguities that can occur regarding the meanings of these various terms the Pontifical Council *Cor Unum* has strongly urged that among Roman Catholics the term 'euthanasia' should be understood to signify its direct active form, and that the term 'passive euthanasia' should be avoided.[159]

Yet even though there can be confusion regarding the meaning of the terms passive and active euthanasia it is still important to draw a distinction between an intention that deliberately sets out

to cause death by an active intervention and the decision to allow
a fatal pathological condition to take its course, culminating in
the death of the patient. To deliberately intervene to kill a patient
would be a violation of the moral principles defended by the
Christian churches. In a terminal case to decide not to continue
treatment is to acknowledge that, for the Christian, death is a
transition rather than a terminus.

Ordinary versus extraordinary means

Moral theologians, whilst taking into account the bias in favour
of human life in Christian theology, have traditionally not seen
physical life as having an absolute value. The inevitability of
death as part of the human condition is enough to show that one
is not obliged, indeed, should not act as if life had to be
prolonged indefinitely. The problem is to find a concrete
criterion where one may let the dying process run its course.

It has been common in Catholic teaching to refer to a
distinction between 'ordinary' and 'extraordinary' means in
answering questions about when a patient is obliged to accept
treatment. In conformity with traditional moral theology certain
contemporary writers have treated this distinction as
synonymous with a distinction between what is obligatory and
what is optional for a particular patient.[160] If it is understood in
this way the distinction clearly needs to be explained by
reference to considerations which are invoked in determining
whether treatment is obligatory. Traditionally moral theology
taught that while extraordinary treatment can permissibly be
forgone, ordinary treatment cannot. Pius XII in his *Discourse on
'reanimation'* of 24 November 1957, follows the distinction of
ordinary and extraordinary, but at once veers away from laying
down a hard and fast line of demarcation. Instead he suggests
that a prudential judgment must be made in concrete cases
taking variable circumstances, such as persons, place, epochs
and culture, into account.[161]

A clear definition of the distinction between ordinary and
extraordinary means is supplied by Paul Ramsey. He writes that
ordinary means of preserving life are all medicines, treatments

and operations, which offer a reasonable hope of benefit for the patient and which can be obtained and used without excessive expense, pain and other inconveniences. Extraordinary means of preserving life are all those medicines, treatments and operations which cannot be obtained without excessive expense, pain or other inconvenience, or which, if used, would not offer a reasonable hope of benefit.[162] Therefore when a treatment was judged by the patient (or by others acting as surrogates) to be excessively burdensome, neither the patient nor surrogate were obliged to begin or continue it. But before a treatment can be considered to be excessively burdensome it is necessary to weigh its burden against whatever benefits it promises. Consequently, it is misleading to suppose that it is possible to compile a specific list of treatments which classifies some as ordinary and others as extraordinary, such that it could help determine whether they should be employed with any particular patient. A treatment that is ordinary for one patient in particular circumstances can be extraordinary for another; or indeed extraordinary for that same patient in different circumstances.

Due to the possibility of ambiguity over the application of these distinctions,[163] numerous criticisms have been levelled against them. Moralists have, therefore, tended to favour terms like 'beneficial', 'non-beneficial', 'excessive burdens' and 'no reasonable hope of recovery'. The traditional starting point for this discussion is the traditional principle of medical ethics: 'to do no harm'. According to W. K. Frankena, this principle of beneficence implies at least the following four things: first, one ought not to inflict evil or harm; second, one ought to prevent evil or harm; third, one ought to remove evil; fourth, one ought to do or promote good.[164] Where it is decided that it is right to inflict injury on patients, it is on the grounds that life and health will be better served by causing the injury—for example, surgery—so that in the long run, pain and suffering will be diminished by this intervention. 'Beneficial means' are not necessarily the same as 'standard treatment' or 'ordinary means'. A good example of this point is given by Sissella Bok: 'Take the case of the person dying of cancer, in great pain, close to death, who develops pneumonia. Certainly antibiotics are now the standard arsenal of medicine; yet many would consider it cruel and extraordinary to use them to prolong such a patient's care.'[165]

The criterion 'excessive burden' has attracted the particular attention of some Roman Catholic theologians. John Connery in a Pope John Center's research study, *Moral Responsibility in Prolonging Life Decisions*, points out that the primary determination of ordinary and extraordinary means rests on this question.[166] The general norm for 'excessive burden' is the common reaction of ordinary people, even though the feelings of some individuals may make the burdens heavier in specific cases.

Theologians include 'great expense' as an index to 'excessive burden', even though health cannot really be measured in terms of money. They simply mean that common sense should judge when an expenditure has become excessive for an individual or family. Today, the public and private reimbursement systems have overshadowed this consideration in certain parts of the world, but it is still a significant factor for many people in developing countries where public health care is minimal and private health insurance is exorbitantly expensive.

The other phrase used to identify an extraordinary means of prolonging life was 'no reasonable hope of recovery'. Connery discusses this concern under the heading of a 'useless' means of prolonging life. In the past, theologians spoke primarily of the uselessness of prolonging terminal illness. This means that a mere prolonging of the dying process can be considered extraordinary.

When addressing the category of a 'useless' means of prolonging life, Fr Gerald Kelly refers to treatments which 'would not offer a reasonable hope of benefit'. Hence he defines extraordinary means as all medicines, treatments and operations which cannot be obtained or used without excessive expense, pain or other inconvenience, or which, if used, would not offer a reasonable hope of benefit.[167] The difficulty lies in attempting to determine the percentage possibility of benefit. A general percentage scale cannot be adhered to because the circumstances of individual patients differ. What is needed is active dialogue between medical practitioners and patients to determine what is considered, in their circumstances, treatment 'without reasonable hope of benefit'.

However, the criterion of 'without reasonable hope of benefit' can be used in an improper way. If a medical treatment successfully accomplishes its purpose, this normally constitutes reasonable hope of benefit. It may be the case that, even after successful treatment, a patient does not enjoy normal health or a normal 'quality of life'. This situation should not be the basis for considering the treatment ethically extraordinary.

Thus, as a matter of principle, the distinction of ordinary and extraordinary means of prolonging life should not be used in a discriminating way against handicapped people. If a medical treatment does not correct one's diminished quality of life, the treatment does not therefore become ethically extraordinary. However, if the medical treatment itself diminishes one's quality of life, it could then be considered ethically extraordinary.[168]

Although the criterion of 'without reasonable hope of benefit' may be used improperly, it applies particularly, but not exclusively, to cases of persons in the final stages of terminal illness. Here, indeed, the 'benefit' may be non-existent if the person is dying a painful death. The Vatican's *Declaration on Euthanasia* in discussing this very situation argues that when inevitable death is imminent in spite of the means used, it is permitted in conscience to take the decision to refuse forms of treatment that would only secure a precarious and burdensome prolongation of life, so long as the normal care due to the sick person in similar cases is not interrupted.[169] Yet it could also be argued that in certain circumstances, although death may not be imminent, it would be permissible to refuse treatment. Take the case of an elderly patient who is diagnosed to have cancer and is offered chemo-therapy. If it can be judged that the treatment would be particularly harsh and debilitating and if it was also unpromising then a decision not to undergo this treatment would be morally permissible.

These reflections on different criteria for judging whether a medical treatment should be considered ethically extraordinary reflect the long and developed Roman Catholic tradition on this matter. A much wider consensus can also be found in both the ethical and medical communities, despite variations of terminology.[170]

A polemical question which arises from this discussion is the one of 'quality of life'. This issue does not concern dying terminal patients but focuses on non-dying terminal patients, or others who, at the price of painful and detrimental interventions, can survive. It is due to the successes of modern medicine and not its failures that society cannot avoid taking into account the quality-of-life dimension.[171] This is due to the fact that certain treatments, although giving a strong probability of success, would make life miserable beyond its true proportion.[172]

There are two quality-of-life criteria relevant to decisions to treat, or to continue treatment or to stop treatment. The first considers the capacity to experience and to relate. According to Richard McCormick, certain treatments do create excessive hardships for an individual and distort and jeopardise their grasp on the overall meaning of life. This is because human relationships, which are the very possibility of growth in love of God and neighbour, would be threatened, strained or submerged so that they would no longer function as the heart and meaning of the individual's life as they should. Something other than the 'higher, more important good' would occupy first place. Life, the condition of other values and achievements, would usurp the place of these and become itself the ultimate value. When that happens, the value of human life has been disrupted out of context.[173]

In *Morals in Medicine*, Thomas O'Donnell develops a similar attitude. While noting that life is a relative, not an absolute good, he poses a question of what it is relative to. In answer to his question he argues that life is the fundamental natural good God has given to people; it is the fundamental context in which all other goods of which God has given to human beings must be exercised. If this is so, then the relativity of the good of life consists in the effort required to preserve this fundamental context and the potentialities of the other goods that still remain to be worked out within that context. Life is therefore, not a value to be preserved in and for itself. To maintain this would commit us to a form of medical vitalism that makes no human or Judeo-Christian sense. It is a value to be preserved precisely as a condition of other values, and therefore insofar as these other values remain attainable. Since these other values cluster around and are rooted in human relationships, it seems to follow that life is a value to be preserved only insofar as it contains some potentiality for human relationships. When one judges this potentiality to be totally absent or because of the condition of the individual, totally subordinate to the mere effort for survival, that life can be said to have achieved its potential.[174]

The second criterion of 'quality of life' considers the intensity of a patient's pain and suffering and his or her susceptibility to treatment. If, despite treatment, there is not and cannot be even a minimal capacity to experience, and to relate, or if the level of pain and suffering will be prolonged, excruciating and intractable, then a decision to cease or not initiate treatment can be preferable to treatment.

It is evident that the word 'life' can mean two things in this context. It can mean a vital or metabolic process, a life incapable of experiencing or communicating and one which therefore could be called 'human biological life'. Or it could mean a level or quality of life which includes both metabolic functions and at least a minimal capacity to experience or communicate which together could be called 'human personal life'.

If by 'life' is meant personal life, then the use of quality-of-life language and criteria need not imply or assume inequality between lives. All persons are equal in value no matter what their condition or quality. But not all lives in the biological sense are of equal value to the patients in question. Death need not always be resisted as if anything is an improvement over death.

One of the more difficult problems in assessing the validity of quality-of-life judgments concerns the definition of the word 'quality'. Because this word is ambiguous, the entire phrase 'quality of life' is subject to expansion to include just about anything, and so its use in medical decision-making is open to serious abuse.[175] This led the editor of the journal *California Medicine* to write that the traditional Western ethic has always placed great emphasis on the intrinsic worth and equal value of every human life regardless of its stage or condition. This traditional ethic is still clearly dominant, but there is much to suggest that it is being eroded at its core and may eventually be abandoned, and in its place emphasis may be laid on something which is beginning to be called the quality of life. So it may become necessary and acceptable to place relative rather than absolute values on such things as human lives, the use of scarce resources and the various elements which are to make up the quality of life or of living which is to be sought.[176]

Opponents of quality-of-life considerations in medical life and death decision-making generally assume the same reductionist and unqualified meaning of quality of life when they characterise it as opposed to or incompatible with sanctity of life. For instance, the theologian Leonard Weber writes that

the quality of life ethic puts the emphasis on the type of life being lived, not upon the fact of life. What the life means to someone is what is important. Keeping this in mind, it is not inappropriate to say that some lives are of greater value than others, that the condition or meaning of life does have much to do with the justification for terminating that life. The sanctity of life ethic defends two propositions. That human life is sacred by the very fact of its existence; its value does not depend upon a certain condition or perfection of that life. That all human lives are of equal value; all have the same right to life. The quality of life ethic finds neither of these two propositions acceptable.[177]

Those who have argued for a sanctity-of-life ethic[178] over and against a quality-of-life ethic are aware that physical life is not an absolute value. On this point they are in total agreement with the proponents of the quality-of-life ethic. However, they maintain that those who support a quality-of-life ethic accord either no value or varying degrees of value to physical life contingent on the presence of some property that life possesses.[179] Such a view, they argue, is intolerable because it denies the equality of physical life and the equality of persons, and thus is a violation of justice. It denies that all lives are inherently valuable, and so some lives can be truly 'not worth living'. Finally, it denies the Christian (especially the Roman Catholic) theological position that human life is valued holistically as body-spirit life by adopting a bi-level anthropology that is committed to sustaining physical life only as an instrumental value.[180] These authors conclude that a sanctity-of-life ethic is superior because it can affirm the equality of life on the grounds that physical life is truly a good or value in itself and not a useful or negotiable value that is dependent on some other intrinsically valuable property.

However, quality-of-life judgments should not be construed as judgments about the value of either physical or personal life. They are not concerned with assessing qualities or properties which, when present, make life itself valuable. Rather, these judgments are evaluative and normative claims or assessments about the relation between the patient's medical condition and the patient's ability to pursue material, moral and spiritual values which transcend physical life but do not give that life its very meaning and worth. As such, they specify concretely the meaning of the terms 'benefits', 'burdens' and 'best interests' of a patient as well as the limits of medical interventions within a given historical and cultural situation.[181]

Thus, when medicine can intervene to ameliorate the quality of the relation between the patient's condition and the pursuit of life's goals, then such an intervention can be considered a benefit to the patient and is in his or her best interests. However, when a proposed intervention cannot offer the patient any reasonable hope for pursuing life's purposes at all because of the condition of the patient; or can only offer the patient a condition where the pursuit of life's purposes will be filled with profound frustration or with utter neglect of these purposes because of the energy needed merely to sustain physical life; then medical interventions can only be a burden to the life treated. In such instances, they are contrary to the best interests of the patient, are harmful to the patient, and medicine having reached its limits on the basis of its own reason for existence should not intervene except to palliate or to comfort the patient.

What becomes clear is that quality-of-life judgments are concerned with what the Vatican *Declaration on Euthanasia* called the assessment of a due proportion between benefits and burdens. However, the proportionality referred to is not about the benefits/burdens of the treatments considered in themselves apart from the patient; rather, the assessment is concerned with the proportionality of benefits/burdens that will affect the quality of the relations between the patient's medical condition and their pursuit of values.[182] With this understanding of 'quality of life' it should be possible to differentiate more accurately between ordinary and extraordinary treatments. The addition of the relational value of life will ensure that a biological essentialism is avoided.

Nutrition and hydration

The moral permissibility of a competent patient, or an incompetent patient's surrogate, deciding to forgo treatments such as respirators or kidney dialysis has become fairly widely accepted by the public and health-care professionals, as well as in recent court decisions. More recently, concern has focused on the provision of artificial nutrition and hydration through the use of nasogastric tubes, intravenous lines, surgically inserted tubes and so forth. The question to be addressed is: Must nutrition and hydration, or food and water, always be continued or may it too permissibly be forgone?

If nutrition and hydration are considered to be medical treatment then the benefits and burdens to the patient of continuing nutrition and hydration as opposed to discontinuing it should be assessed. For nearly all patients that assessment will favour continuing them, but in a few cases it need not do so.[183] The process of providing nutrition and hydration can itself involve substantial ineliminable burdens for patients. For example, in cases where patients' diseases makes absorbing nutrition the cause of significant discomfort or where patients' dementia and resultant confusion requires physical restraint to prevent their removing the feeding tubes. In a very few other cases, the quality of the life given by continued nutrition and hydration may be substantially and unalterably burdensome to patients. For most patients, discontinuing nutrition and hydration would result in substantial subjective distress and would very likely not be in their interests, even if death might otherwise be welcome to them.[184]

This conclusion is challenged on the traditional grounds that a patient's refusal of food and drink is suicide and therefore wrong, and on the grounds that life is a gift from God and a person is not at liberty to destroy it. However, a further concern about permitting the forgoing of nutrition and hydration centres on its symbolic effect together with worries about abuse.[185] The provision of food and water is one of the very first acts of concern and support each person receives as he or she enters the world. Throughout life, feeding the hungry is invested with great moral importance, and starvation is associated with suffering and strong moral repugnance. Society should be reluctant to weaken this concern by permitting suffering or death from starvation. This is especially so since many of those who might be endangered by any weakening of the requirement to provide food and water are debilitated and vulnerable, unable to protect themselves and to assert their own interests. Permitting the withholding of food and water risks the deliberate killing of the vulnerable and burdensome on morally unacceptable grounds such as the economic costs of sustaining their lives. Moreover, many see any withholding of food and water as only a small step to euthanasia in all its forms.[186]

Within the Roman Catholic Church different episcopal conferences have taken different views regarding the morality of removing nutrition and hydration from the permanent comatose and patients in persistent vegetative states (PVS). The Washington bishops, joined by the bishops in Oregon, address the question of the care of the irreversibly comatose or persistent vegetative patient in a pastoral letter entitled *Living and Dying Well*.[187] They acknowledge that 'conscientious Catholic moral theologians and many others in our society have not achieved consensus about this point'.[188] Given the lack of agreement on the issues, the Washington and Oregon bishops hold that 'decisions regarding artificial administered nutrition and hydration must be made on a case-by-case basis, in light of the benefits and burdens they entail for the individual patient', and then conclude: 'In appropriate circumstances, the decision to withhold these means of life support can be in accord with Catholic moral reasoning and ought to be respected by medical care givers and the laws of the land.'[189]

This position is at odds with the Catholic bishops of Massachusetts, who insist 'the authentic teaching of the Catholic Church' requires that 'nutrition and hydration should always be provided [to irreversibly comatose patients] when they are capable of sustaining life'.[190] The Pennsylvania bishops argue that withdrawal of artificial nutrition-hydration involves, in most cases, the intent to kill: it is murder by omission. The PVS patient is not in a terminal condition. It is only if nutrition-hydration is removed that the patient will die. 'It is the removal of the nutrition and hydration that brings about the death.' This is not merely 'allowing to die'. The bishops believe it involves the clear intent to bring about death.

The view of these bishops finds support from a group of ethicists (including William May, Germain Grisez, William Smith, Mark Siegler, Robert Barry and Orville Griese) who, writing in *Issues in Law and Medicine*, argued that in their 'judgment, feeding such patients [who are permanently unconscious] and providing them with fluids by means of tubes is not useless in the strict sense, because it does bring to these patients a great benefit, namely, the preservation of their lives'.[191] They go on to note that the damage or debilitating condition of the patient has been the key factor in recent court cases and conclude that decisions to withdraw food have been made 'because sustaining life was judged to be of no benefit to a person in such poor condition. These demands, they conclude, have been unjust.'

In the ethical discussion of artificial nutrition and hydration for patients in a persistent vegetative state, many philosophers and theologians have concluded that the provision of such nutrition and hydration is not morally mandatory because it can no longer benefit the patient.[192] This understanding has also been accepted by many courts and several medical groups[193] which have approved such withdrawal. It has also been approved by the United States President's Commission for the Study of Ethical Problems in Medicine and Biomedical and Behavioral Research.

This view has found support from bio-ethicists such as Dennis Brodeur, Kevin O'Rourke, Albert Moraczewski, John Paris, James Walter, James Bresnahan, Daniel Callahan, Albert Jonsen and Thomas Shannon. According to Dennis Brodeur, artificial nutrition-hydration that 'simply puts off death by maintaining physical existence with no hope of recovery . . . is useless and therefore not ethically obligatory'.[194] According to Kevin O'Rourke 'withholding artificial hydration and nutrition from a patient in an irreversible coma does not induce a new fatal pathology; rather it allows an already existing fatal pathology to take its natural course'. Therefore O'Rourke argues that this is not a discussion on whether death is imminent, but 'whether a fatal pathology is present'. If it is, the key moral question is 'whether there is a moral obligation to seek to remove the fatal pathology or at least to circumvent its effects'.[195] He goes on to state that by definition, a patient in an irreversible coma cannot eat and swallow and thus will die of that pathology in a short time unless life-prolonging devices are utilised to circumvent the pathology.[196] Therefore, those who argue that death is caused by withdrawing nutrition and hydration are actually introducing a new cause of death and have overlooked the lethal causal character of the underlying pathology.[197]

This emphasises the central issue in this debate, namely the notion of benefit. William May sees nutrition and hydration for a PVS patient as providing a 'great benefit', the preservation of life. O'Rourke believes that mere 'physical function bereft of the potential for cognitive-affect function does not benefit the patient' and is, in this sense, useless. The goal of medical treatment is 'not merely to cause an effect on some portion of the patient's anatomy, physiology or chemistry, but to benefit the patient as a whole'. Nutritional support can effectively preserve a host of organ systems of a PVS patient but remain futile. Because 'the ultimate goal of any treatment should be improvement of the patient's prognosis, comfort, well-being or general state of health. A treatment that fails to provide such a benefit—even though it produces a measurable effect—should be considered futile.'[198]

In a similar debate within the United Kingdom the Law Lords' decision to allow the doctors to withdraw nutrition and hydration from Anthony Bland who was in a persistent vegetative state due to being crushed in a football stadium disaster provoked a sharp response from the Joint Committee on Bio-Ethical Issues, of the Catholic Bishops of England, Ireland, Scotland and Wales. They state that the judgment of the Law Lords in the case of Airedale NHS Hospital Trust v. Bland seriously erodes both recognition of the principle of respect for the sanctity of human life and the legal protection owing to innocent and vulnerable human beings, particularly those in the care of doctors. They point out that the Law Lords accepted the proposition that those who have the care of patients in a condition such as the judges described in the case of Anthony Bland may rightly adopt a pattern of care with the intention, purpose or aim[199] of terminating the lives or bringing about the deaths of those patients. That is a proposition which the Catholic Church formally rejects, and which is incompatible with the moral and legal norms which have hitherto held sway in our civilisation. While noting the Catholic teaching on treatment and the debate about the classification of tube feeding, they state that it can never be morally acceptable to withdraw tube feeding precisely to end a patient's life.[200]

Anthony Fisher in supporting the bishops' position argues that the major issue in the Bland case was whether tube-feeding should be considered as 'medical treatment' which could be viewed, in certain circumstances, as extraordinary. The Catholic Church authorities have repeatedly said it is not,[201] although theologians are divided on the issue.[202] He argues that in tube-feeding there are two separate issues. The first is the feeding-tube itself while the second is the provision of food through the feeding tube. A feeding-tube should be viewed in the same light as a tracheal tube which allows some patients to breathe, or a catheter which allows them to pass water. The tube itself is entirely passive once inserted although its insertion might be regarded as medical treatment and its maintenance as nursing care. Once inserted it allows a natural bodily function to take place, rather than actively taking them over. Fisher argues that if we consider the provision of food through such a feeding-tube as medical treatment then so is allowing or providing air through a tracheal tube and draining urine through a catheter. Clean air, food, water, clothing and sanitation are needs of any persons, well or ill. The giving of them merely provides for these basic, universal needs. When given to a dependent person, they are about as basic a kind of care as we can give, the bottom line of any active expression of equal concern and respect. Just as we do not define hunger and thirst as pathologies or clinical conditions, so we do not normally define the giving of food and water as treatments, even if it requires some medical assistance. Giving food and water is not aimed at preventing or curing illness, retarding deterioration, or relieving pain and suffering. Thus unlike 'medical treatment, as it is ordinarily understood, no consent is required when providing clothing, shelter, hygienic and sanitary care, nutrition and fluids in a medical context'. He goes on to say that even if tube-feeding is regarded as 'medical treatment' or part of a whole regime of medical and nursing care, it cannot properly be regarded as 'extraordinary' or optional care, since it is neither futile nor is its provision generally overly burdensome.[203]

This position did not gain general acceptance in Catholic circles in England. Kevin Kelly in referring to moralists such as Gerald Kelly and Edwin Healy[204] writes that he has no doubt that the permanent use of medical nutrition and hydration in the case of Tony Bland was extraordinary, and so an optional means of sustaining his life, 'in which case they would have insisted that ethically its withdrawal was not an instance of killing by starvation'. He goes on to state that these writers would have strongly defended the moral legitimacy of the decision taken by Tony's parents and his doctor.[205] As additional support for his arguments he refers to Kevin O'Rourke, whose position we have already examined and the Catholic bishops of Texas. They arrive at a similar conclusion when they write that the morally appropriate forgoing or withdrawing of artificial nutrition and hydration from a permanently unconscious person is not abandoning that person. Rather, it is accepting the fact that the person has come to the end of his or her pilgrimage and should not be impeded from taking the final step.[206]

The decision of whether to maintain or withdraw artificial nutrition and hydration is an extremely complex issue. How a decision is arrived at will, in part, be determined by how artificial nutrition and hydration is understood. If it is viewed as ordinary care which society is obliged to offer all its citizens then its withdrawal from persistently vegetative patients becomes ethically problematic. However, if in certain circumstances it is perceived to be medical treatment which is delaying a fatal pathology from taking its normal course then it can be understood to be extraordinary care. If within a given set of circumstances this is found to be the case the removal of artificial nutrition and hydration could be morally acceptable. When decisions of this sort are made not only does the extraordinariness of the treatment need to be assessed but also whether this treatment is beneficial or non-beneficial to the patient and what quality of life it enhances.

It is evident that the issues of passive and active euthanasia, ordinary and extraordinary means, and artificial nutrition and hydration are complex and no widespread consensus exists on them as yet. According to Dan Brock there is, however, a central core of widespread agreement. A competent patient, or an incompetent patient's surrogate, is ethically entitled to assess the benefits and burdens of any proffered treatment according to the patient's own aims and values and to accept or reject the treatment. The quite broad agreement on this seemingly simple principle should in no way be taken to imply, however, that the decisions themselves in concrete cases are simple or uncontroversial for those involved in them. There is much truth in the view that the particular circumstances and details of each case make it unique. No simple principles can be mechanically applied in a way that makes for easy choices. Decisions about life and death are inevitably and quite properly difficult and troubling and require sensitive, thoughtful and wise judgments from all involved.[207] The way forward in the euthanasia debate appears to be the attempt to arrive at a balance between the fundamental value of life and the relational dimension of human living which ensures the fulfilment of this value.

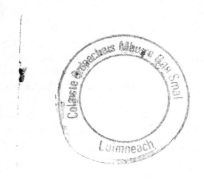

NOTES

Introduction (pages vii–xii)
1. *The Tablet*, 9 October 1993, 1309.

Chapter 1 (pages 1–57)
1. The word 'abortion' comes from the Latin word *aboriri*, meaning 'to fail to be born'.
2. The English and American spellings of 'foetus' and 'fetus' differ. Etymologists and anatomists agree that 'fetus' is the correct usage as the word is derived from the Latin *feto*—I bear. However, English clinicians still insist on using the word 'foetus'. In this study the word 'fetus' will be used unless cited in a quotation.
3. *Moscow Business Times*, September 1992.
4. In 1990 there were 186,912 abortions in England and Wales; of these over 60,000 were performed under 9 weeks; 85,000 between 9–12 weeks; 21,000 between 13–19 weeks; and about 2,000 from 20 weeks and over. Of the 186,912 abortions in 1990 the following was the age of the mother at termination: under 15: 1,000; 15: 3,000; 16–19: 39,000; 20–24: 58,000; 25–29: 41,000; 30–34: 23,000; 35–39: 12,000; 40–44: 5,000; 45 and over: 900. 113,330 abortions were performed in non-National Health Service hospitals and 73,582 in National Health Service hospitals.
5. M. Potts, P. Diggory and J. Peel, *Abortion* (Cambridge: Cambridge University Press, 1977), 108–9.
6. D. Callahan, *Abortion: Law, Choice and Morality* (New York: Macmillan, 1972), 246.
7. Ibid., 294.
8. Ibid., 202–3.
9. K. Janmejai, 'Socio-Economic Aspects of Abortion', *Family Planning News, India* 4 (1963), 55.
10. B. Hutchinson, 'Induced Abortion in Brazilian Married Women', *America Latina* 7 (1964), 21.
11. W. L. Langer, 'Europe's Initial Population Explosion', *American Historical Review* 69 (1963), 1.

12. M. Potts, op. cit., 114.
13. R. Armijo and T. Monteal, 'The Problem of Induced Abortion in Chile', *Midbank Memorial Fund Quarterly* 43 (1965), 265.
14. D. Callahan, op. cit., 297.
15. M. Potts, op. cit., 118.
16. Justice Lane, *Report of the Committee on the Working of the Abortion Act*, vol. III (London: HMSO, 1974), 35.
17. J. Noonan, 'An Almost Absolute Value in History', in *The Morality of Abortion: Legal and Historical Perspectives*. Edited by J. Noonan (Cambridge, Mass: Harvard University Press, 1977), 4.
18. J. Noonan, *Contraception: A History of its Treatment by the Catholic Theologians and Canonists* (Cambridge, Mass: Harvard University Press, 1965), 18–29.
19. H. E. Sigerist, *A History of Medicine*, vol. 1 (Oxford: Oxford University Press, 1951), 430.
20. Exodus 21:22–5. From *The Revised English Bible*.
21. *The Septuagint Version of the Old Testament an Apocrypha*, in *Christian Classics* (Westminster: Zondervan Publishing, 1975).
22. J. Connery, *Abortion: The Development of the Roman Catholic Perspective* (USA: Loyola University Press, 1975), 17.
23. G. R. Dunstan, 'The Human Embryo in the Western Moral Tradition', in *The Status of the Human Embryo*. Edited by G. R. Dunstan and M. Seller (London: King Edward's Hospital Fund of London, 1988), 41–3.
24. B. Häring, *Medical Ethics* (Slough: St Paul's Publications, 1972), 98–9.
25. J. Noonan, 'An Almost Absolute Value in History', op. cit., 9.
26. *The Didache*, 2:2, see J. Noonan, 'An Almost Absolute Value in History', op. cit., 9.
27. It is not known who Barnabas was, but it is certain that he was not the apostle of that name. Some think he was an Alexandrian. His Epistle, like the Didache, was an attempt to explain the demands of Christian life to prospective converts from paganism.
28. J. Connery, op. cit., 36.
29. In Aristotle's usage the term soul (*psyche*) or animating principle (from the Latin *anima*) was that which gave to a substance or organism its characteristic form.
30. N. Ford, *When Did I Begin?* (Cambridge: Cambridge University Press, 1989), 28.
31. *Apologia*, 9.8, CSEL 64:25. The ancients knew nothing about the female ovum, and hence nothing about fertilisation.

Conception occurred when the semen was planted in the uterus. The most common opinion, that of Aristotle, considered the semen the active agent in generation. The *Catamenia* (menstrual blood) of the woman provided the matter of generation. See *On Generation of Animals,* 1, 19–20, *Works of Aristotle*, 5:727–8.

32. *De Anima* c 25 section 4. *Ante-Nicene Christian Library* vol. 15, 470.
33. The destruction of the fetus by dismemberment.
34. The deliberate crushing of the fetus's skull.
35. *Ep 188 Ad Amphilochium II* PG 32:671.
36. *Adversus Macedonianos.*
37. *Quaestionum in Hepttateuchum*, 1 11 no. 80.
38. G. R. Dunstan, op. cit., 45.
39. *Summa Theologica* 2.2.64.8.
40. That a being does not have a rational soul at conception formed a principal objection for him to the doctrine of the Immaculate Conception of Mary, which he denied, *In Libros IV Sententiarum* 3.1.1: she was 'sanctified' in the womb, but 'when it definitely was, is uncertain'.
41. J. Noonan, op. cit., 23.
42. C. Means, 'A Historical View', in *Abortion in a Changing World*, vol. 1. Edited by Robert Hall (New York: Columbia University Press, 1970), 20.
43. J. Noonan, op. cit., 26.
44. Sanchez, *De Sancto Matrimonii Sacramento* at 9.20.9.
45. C. Means, op. cit., 19.
46. J. Noonan, op. cit., 32.
47. Gratian it appears had three sources from which to draw: the early canons, the penitential books, and the Fathers. Curiously he made use neither of the early canons nor of the penitential books, but only of the Fathers. The source of the basic thesis he chose on abortion was the *Decretum* of the *Panormia* of Ivo of Chartres. See J. Connery, op. cit., 90ff.
48. D. Callahan, op. cit., 412.
49. J. Noonan, op. cit., 32–3.
50. *Bullarium diplomatum et privilegiorum*, 9:39–42.
51. *Bullarium*, 9:431.
52. *Ineffabilis Deus*, Denzinger at 1641.
53. J. Noonan, op. cit., 38.
54. *Acta apostolicae sedis*, 5.298 (1869).
55. *Codex Iuris Canonici* c. 2350, 1.
56. *Codex Iuris Canonici (CIC)*, c. 1398.
57. *CIC*, no 1398.

58. *CIC*, no. 1314.
59. *CIC*, nos. 1323–4.
60. *Catechism of the Universal Church* (Dublin: Veritas, 1994), no. 2272 at 489.
61. Pius XI, *Cast connubii, Acta Apostolicae Sedis* 22.562 (1930).
62. Ibid., at 563.
63. Ibid., at 564.
64. From *Papal Teachings: The Human Body* (Boston: St Paul Editions, 1960), 60.
65. Pius XII, *Acta Apostolicae Sedis*, 43:838–9 (1951).
66. *Acta Apostolicae Sedis*, 53 (1961), 401.
67. *Gaudium et spes*, no. 51. In A. Flannery, (ed), *Vatican Council II: The Conciliar and Post Conciliar Documents* (Dublin: Dominican Publications, 1981), 954–5.
68 B. Häring in Vorgrimler (ed), *Commentary Documents of Vatican II*, vol. V, 243.
69. Paul VI, *Humanae Vitae*, 25 July 1968. In *Acta Apostolicae Sedis*, 60 (1968), 481.
70. Congregation for the Doctrine of the Faith, *Declaration on Procured Abortion (Questio de abortu)*, 18 November 1974, no. 12. In A. Flannery, (ed), *Vatican Council Documents: More Post Conciliar Documents*, vol. 2 (Dublin: Dominican Publications, 1982), 445–6.
71. *Declaration on Procured Abortion*, op. cit., no. 13.
72. Apostolic See, *Chapter of the Rights of the Family*, Art 4. 23 October 1983.
73. M. Coughlin, *The Vatican, the Law and the Human Embryo* (London: Macmillan, 1990), 65. Italics mine.
74. Romans 8:15–22.
75. *Redemptor hominis*, 11.8.
76. *Dives in misericordia*, 11.2.
77. *Veritatis splendor*, no. 80.
78. John Paul II, Homily given in Washington DC at Capital Hill on 7 October 1979.
79. *Catechism*, op. cit., no. 2270, at 489. Refer Congregation for the Doctrine of the Faith, *Donum Vitae*, 22 February 1987 (Dublin: Veritas, 1987), no. I.1.
80. *Catechism*, op. cit., no. 2273, at 489.
81. *Donum Vitae*, III.
82. *The Tablet*, 1 April 1995, 432.
83. Pope John Paul II, *Evangelium Vitae* (Vatican City: Libreria Editrice Vaticana, 1995), no. 52, 93.
84. Ibid., no. 57, 101.

85. Ibid., no. 58, 104.

86. Ibid., no. 58, 105.

87. Ibid., no. 62, 112.

88. Ibid., no. 62. 113.

89. Editorial, *The Daily Telegraph*, 31 March 1995, 26.

90. P. Ramsey, 'The Morality of Abortion', in *Life or Death: Ethics and Options* (Seattle: University of Washington Press, 1968), 72.

91. Ibid., 73.

92. J. Fuchs, *Natural Law*, trans. H. Reckter and J. Dowling (New York: Sheed and Ward, 1965), 65. See also D. Granfield, *The Abortion Decision* (New York: Doubleday, 1969), 126.

93. N. St John-Stevas, *The Right to Life* (New York: Holt, Rinehart and Winston, 1964), 12.

94. Ibid., 17.

95. See B. Häring, *The Law of Christ*, vol. III (Westminster, Maryland: Newman Press, 1965), 194; D. Cairns, *God Up There?* (Philadelphia: Westminster Press, 1967), 27.

96. D. Callahan, op. cit., 311.

97. R. A. McCormick, 'Morality of War', in *New Catholic Encyclopedia* (New York: McGraw-Hill, 1967), vol. 14, 805.

98. N. Ford, op. cit., 57.

99. *Declaration on Procured Abortion*, op. cit., no. 12, 445–6.

100. This declaration expressly leaves aside the question of the moment when the spiritual soul is infused. There is not a unanimous tradition on this point and authors are as yet in disagreement. For some it dates from the first instant, for others it could not at least precede nidation. It is not within the competence of science to decide between these views, because the existence of an immortal soul is not a question in its field. It is a philosophical problem from which our moral affirmation remains independent for two reasons: (i) supposing a later animation, there is still nothing less than a *human* life, preparing for and calling for a soul in which the nature received from parents is completed; (ii) on the other hand it suffices that this presence of the soul be probable (and one can never prove the contrary) in order that the taking of life involves accepting the risk of killing a man, not only waiting for, but already in possession of his soul. *Declaration on Procured Abortion*, op. cit., no. 19, 452.

101. N. Ford, op. cit., 62–4.

102. R. A. McCormick, *Notes on Moral Theology: 1965 through 1980* (University Press of America, 1981), 515.

103. See H. Noldin, A. Schmitt, and G. Heinzel, *Summa Theologiae Moralis* I (31st ed.; Innsbruck: F. Rauch, 1956), 84ff.

104. *Acta Apostolicae Sedis*, 43 (1951), 855.
105. A. Bouscaren, *Ethics of Ectopic Operations* (Milwaukee: Bruce, 1943), 1–2.
106. C. Van Der Poel, 'The Principle of Double Effect', *Absolutes in Moral Theology*. Edited by Charles Curran (Washington, DC: Corpus Books, 1968), 204–5.
107. D. Callahan, op. cit., 424.
108. J. Gustafson, 'A Protestant Ethical Approach', in *The Morality of Abortion*, op. cit., 102–6.
109. J. Donceel, 'Abortion: Mediated vs Immediate Animation', *Continuum*, vol. V (1967), 167–71. Cf. Donceel, 'A Liberal Catholic View', *Abortion in a Changing World*. Edited by R. E. Hall (New York: Columbia University Press, 1970), vol. 1, 39–45.
110. J. Donceel, *Theological Studies* vol. XXXI (1970), 83, 101.
111. J. Donceel, 'A Liberal Catholic View', *The Problem of Abortion*. Edited by Joel Feinbery (Belmont, California: Wadeworth, 1984), 15.
112. J. Mahoney, *Bioethics and Belief* (London: Sheed and Ward, 1984), 66–7.
113. N. Ford, op. cit., 181–2.
114. N. Ford, op. cit., 176–7.
115. Jacques-Marie Pohier, 'Reflexions theologiques sur la position de l'eglise catholique', *Lumiere et Vie*, vol. XXI, no. 109 (Aout–Octobre, 1972), 84.
116. Louis Beinart, 'L'avortement est-il infanticide?,' *Etudes*, vol. CCCXXXIII (1970), 522.
117. B. Ribes, 'Recherche philosophique et theologique', *Avortement et respect de la vie humaine*, 202.
118. B. Quelquejeu, 'La volonte de procreer', *Lumiere et Vie*, vol. XXI, no. 109 (Aout–Octobre, 1972), 57–62.
119. B. Häring, *Medical Ethics* (Notre Dame, IN: Fides, 1973), 89.
120. R. McCormick, 'Rules for Abortion Debate', in *Abortion: the Moral Issues*. Edited by E. Batchelor (New York: Pilgrim Press, 1982), 35.
121. C. Curran, *A New Look at Christian Morality* (Notre Dame, IN: Fides, 1968), 243.
122. B. Häring, *Free and Faithful in Christ*, vol. 3 (Middlegreen, Slough: St Paul Publications, 1982), 33.
123 Ibid., 34.
124. B. Häring, *Shalom: Peace. The Sacrament of Reconciliation* (New York: Farrar, Strauss and Giroux, 1968), 181.
125. B. Häring, 'A Theological Evaluation', in *The Morality of*

Abortion: Legal and Historical Perspectives. Edited by John Noonan (London: Harvard University Press, 1977), 140–43.

126. G. Baum, 'Abortion: An Ecumenical Dilemma', in *Abortion: The Moral Issues.* Edited by E. Batchelor (New York: Pilgrim Press, 1982), 42–3.

127. P. Simmons, 'A Theological Response to Fundamentalism on the Abortion Issue', in *Abortion: the Moral Issues*, op. cit., 175–6.

128. B. Waltke, 'Reflections from the Old Testament on Abortion', *Presidential Address at the December 29, 1975, Meeting of the Evangelical Theological Society*, 11.

129. P. Simmons, op. cit., 180.

130. J. Stott, 'Reverence for Human Life', *Christianity Today*, vol. XVI, no. 18 (9 June 1972), 12.

131. Not all fundamentalists agree on this. Bruce Waltke, for instance uses the notion of the biological transmission of sin to argue that the fetus is a sinner by conception and thus a person.

132. See previous section for a full analysis of this text.

133. The US situation was different in that no new legislation was introduced. The liberalisation of the law was due to a reinterpretation of the 14th Amendment by the Supreme Court. For a full analysis of both British and American abortion legislation see M. Potts, P. Diggory and J. Peel, *Abortion* (Cambridge: Cambridge University Press, 1977).

134. *Population Trends* no. 64, Summer 1991, HMSO.

135. Cf. K. Kelly, *Life and Live* (London: Collins, 1987), 52.

136. Board of Social Responsibility of the Church of Scotland: *Study Group on Abortion and Report on Warnock Report*, in *Reports to the General Assembly*, 1985, 283.

137. Ibid., 284–5.

138. K. Boyd, B. Callaghan and E. Shotter, *Life Before Birth* (London: SPCK, 1986), 104.

139. Board of Social Responsibility of the Church of Scotland, *Reports to the General Assembly*, 1987, 1988, 277.

140. Ibid., 276–7.

141. Ibid.

142. *Abortion: An Ethical Discussion* (London: CIO Publishing, 1965), 61–2.

143. J. Habgood, 'Euthanasia—A Christian View', *Journal of the Royal Society of Health* 3 (1974): 124, 126.

144. A Report by the Board for Social Responsibility, *Abortion and the Church: What are the Issues?* (London: Church House Publishing, 1993), 27.

145. Ibid., 25–6.

146. Ibid., 26.
147. Methodist Conference, 'The Methodist Statement on Abortion 1976', in *Status of the Unborn Human* (Peterborough: Methodist Publishing House, 1990), 51.
148. Ibid., 51–2.
149. Ibid., 52.
150. K. Kelly, op. cit., 61.
151. Methodist Conference, *Status of the Unborn Human* (Peterborough: Methodist Publishing House, 1990), 33.
152. This is a genetically inherited disease affecting the haemoglobin of the blood and is a common cause of stillbirth in South East Asia. There is no known cure and the defect is always fatal.
153. Methodist Conference, *Status of the Unborn Human*, op. cit., 34–6.
154. K. Barth, 'The Protection of Life', in *Abortion: the Moral Issues*, op. cit., 95.
155. Ibid., 97.
156. Ibid., 98–9.
157. Ibid., 101.
158. This was the case which appeared before the US Supreme Court and led to a reinterpretation of the 14th Amendment.
159. P. Ramsey, 'The Morality of Abortion', in *The Ethics of Abortion*. Edited by R. Baird and S. Rosenbaum, (Buffalo: Prometheus Books, 1989), 61 & 66.
160. R. Dworkin, *Life's Dominion: An Argument about Abortion and Euthanasia* (London: HarperCollins, 1993), 39.
161. Cf. R. Dworkin, 36–7.
162. Ibid., 37.
163. James Gustafson, 'A Protestant Ethical Approach', in *The Morality of Abortion: Legal and Historical Perspectives*. Edited by J. Noonan (London: Harvard University Press, 1977), 116.
164. R. Bainton, *Christian Attitudes toward War and Peace* (New York: Abingdon Press, 1960), 98.
165. J. Gustafson, op. cit., 122.
166. R. McCormick, *Notes on Moral Theology: 1964 through 1980* (University Press of America, 1981), 500–501.
167. R. F. Gardner, *Abortion: the Personal Dilemma* (London: Exeter, 1972), 126.
168. Ibid., 123.
169. Ibid., 123.
170. Ibid., 131.
171. N. Cameron and P. Sims, 'Defending Abortion', *Ethics and Medicine* 2:3 (1986), 38.

172. K. Kelly, op. cit., 65.
173. Ibid., 75–6.
174. B. Häring, *Free and Faithful in Christ*, vol. 3, op. cit., 34.

Chapter 2 (pages 58–122)

1. The generation of fully mature ova (the process is called oogenesis) involves several cell divisions with special names for each of the several developing cells. For simplicity, the term 'egg' will be used in following the cells that become the mature ovum through all its developmental stages.

2. Chromosomes are the threads within the nucleus of a cell which become visible during cell division. They occur in pairs—one member of maternal and one of paternal origin. They are regarded today as the major carriers of genetic material, consisting of DNA and various types of protein. The position of a particular gene on a chromosome is called its *locus*. A normal human body cell has 46 chromosomes: 22 pairs of autosomes together with (in females) one matching pair of X chromosomes and (in males) one non-matching pair, the X and Y chromosome.

3. L. Kaplan and C. Kaplan, 'Natural Reproduction and Reproduction-Aiding Technologies', in *The Ethics of Reproductive Technology*. Edited by K. Alpern (Oxford: Oxford University Press, 1992), 18–19.

4. Infertility is not necessarily permanent or untreatable, in contrast to sterility, which is irreversible by therapeutic intervention, as in the case of a woman who lacks ovaries or a man who lacks testes. On infertility and sterility generally see: D. Epel, 'The Program of Fertilization', *Scientific American* 237 (1977): 128–38 and 'Fertilization', *Endeavour* (New Series), 4 (1980), 26–31.

5. US Congress, Office of Technological Assessment, *Reproductive Hazards in the Workplace*, OTA–BA–266 (Washington, DC: US Government Printing Office, December 1985).

6. L. Kaplan and C. Kaplan, op. cit., 20.

7. M. Mazor, 'Barren Couples', *Psychology Today* 12 (May 1979), 101, 103–4, 107–8, 110.

8. M. Mazor, 'Emotional Reactions to Infertility', in *The Ethics of Reproductive Technology*. Edited by K. Alpern (Oxford: Oxford University Press, 1992), 33.

9. B. Menning, *Infertility: A Guide for the Childless Couple* (Englewood Cliffs, New Jersey: Prentice-Hall, 1977).

10. H. Walker, 'Sexual Problems and Infertility', *Psychosomatic* 19 (1978), 477–87.

11. C. Debrovner and R. Shubin-Stein, 'Sexual Problems Associated with Infertility', *Medical Aspects of Human Sexuality* 10 (March 1976), 161–2.
12. M. Mazor, 'Emotional Reactions to Infertility', op. cit., 34.
13. Ibid., 37–8.
14. M. Talmor, *Infertility* (New York: Grune and Stratton, 1978).
15. J. Yeh and M. Seibel, 'Artificial Insemination with Donor Sperm: A Review of 108 Patients', *Obstet Gynecol* 70 (1987), 313–16.
16. M. Vekemans, et al, 'In Vitro Fertilization with donor sperm after failure of artificial insemination', *Human Reproduction* 2 (1987), 121–5.
17. L. Andrews, 'The Stock Market: The Law and New Reproductive Technologies', *American Bar Association* 70 (1984), 50–56.
18. Refer to *Warnock Committee Report*.
19. C. Grobstein, 'External Human Fertilization', *Scientific American* 240 (1979), 57–67; P. C. Steptoe and R. G. Edwards, 'Laparoscopic Recovery of Preovulatory Human Oocytes after Priming of Ovaries with Gonadotropins', *The Lancet* 1 (1970), 683–9; M. Gold, 'The Baby Makers', *Science* 85 6 (April 1985), 26–8.
20. P. Dellenbach, et al, 'Transvaginal Sonographically Controlled Follicle Puncture for Oocyte Retrieval', *Fertilization Sterilization* 44 (1985), 656.
21. L. Kaplan and C. Kaplan, op. cit., 26.
22. D. McLaughlin, 'A Scientific Introduction to Reproductive Technologies', in *Reproductive Technologies, Marriage and the Church*. Edited by the Pope John Center (Braintree, Mass: Pope John Center, 1988), 59.
23. Ibid., 64–5.
24. L. Andrews, *New Conception* (New York: St Martin's Press, 1984), 243–66; J. Treichel, 'Embryo Transfers Achieved in Humans', *Science News* 124 (1983), 69.
25. Human Fertilisation and Embryology Authority (HFEA), *Donated Ovarian Tissue in Embryo Research and Assisted Conception: Public Consultation Document* (London: Human Fertilisation and Embryology Authority, 1994), 3.
26. Ky Cha et al, 'Pregnancy after in vitro fertilization of human follicular oocytes collected from non-stimulated cycles, their culture in vitro and their transfer in a donor oocyte program', *Fertility and Sterility* 55 (1991), 109–13.
27. R. T. Morris, 'The Ovarian Graft', *New York Medical Journal* 62 (1985), 436.

28. W. Russell and P. Douglas, 'Offspring from unborn mothers', *Proceedings of the National Academy of Sciences, USA* 31 (1945), 402–4.

29. HFEA, op. cit., 4.

30. D. Fletcher, 'Aborted foetuses cannot be used to help childless', *Daily Telegraph*, 21 July 1994, 7.

31. J. Laurance, 'Ban on using foetal ovaries to treat childless', *The Times*, 21 July 1994, 6.

32. R. H. Glass and R. J. Ericisson, 'Sex Selection', in *Getting Pregnant in the 1980s*, 113–28; and R. H. Blank, *Redefining Human Life: Reproduction Technologies and Social Policy* (Boulder, Co: Westview Press, 1984), 68–70.

33. L. Kaplan, and C. Kaplan, op. cit., 28–9.

34. Legislation to limit experimentation was enacted in Ontario in 1985, the United Kingdom in 1984; by the United States Ethics Advisory Board in 1979, and in Australia in 1984.

35. DNA or Deoxyribonucleic Acid. The nucleic acid which occurs in combination with protein in the chromosomes, and which contains the genetic instructions. It consists of four primary nitrogenous bases (adenine, guanine, thymine and cytosine), a sugar (2-deoxy-D-ribose), and phosphoric acid, arranged in a regular structure. The skeleton of the DNA consists of two chains of alternate sugar and phosphate groups twisted round each other in the form of a double spiral, or double helix; to each sugar is attached a base; and the two chains are held together by hydrogen bonding between the bases. The sequence of bases provides in code the genetic information. Each human cell nucleus contains approximately 6x109 base pairs of DNA, totalling in length about 2m/6.6ft, but coiled upon itself again and again, that it fits inside the cell nucleus. DNA replicates itself accurately during cell growth and duplication, and its structure is stable, so that heritable changes (mutations) are very infrequent.

36. M. Ferguson, 'Contemporary and Future Possibilities for Human Embryonic Manipulation', in *Experiments on Embryos*. Edited by A. Dyson and J. Harris (London: Routledge, 1990), 7–8.

37. The most likely genes to be used in the first experiment on human gene therapy are: *Hypoxanthine-Guanine Phosphoribosyl Transferase (PHRT)*, the absence of which results in *Lesch-Nyhan Disease*—a severe neurological disorder which includes uncontrollable self-mutilation; *Adenosine Deaminase (ADA)*, the absence of which results in severe immunodeficiency disease—in which children have a greatly

weakened resistance to infection and cannot survive the usual childhood diseases; and *Purine Nucleo-Side Phosphorylase (PNP)* the absence of which results in another severe form of immunodeficiency disease. For all three, the clinical syndrome is profoundly debilitating. Refer W. French Anderson, 'Human Gene Therapy: Scientific and Ethical Considerations', in *Ethics, Reproduction and Genetic Control*. Edited by R. Chadwick (London: Routledge, 1987), 148.

38. T. Wilkie, *Perilous Knowledge: The Human Genome Project and Its Implications* (London: Faber and Faber, 1993), 151.
39. *The Lancet.* Cited by W. Bodmer and R. McKie, *The Book of Man: The Quest to Discover Our Genetic Heritage* (London: Little, Brown and Company, 1994), 244.
40. W. French Anderson. Cited by W. Bodmer and R. McKie, op. cit., 244.
41. T. Wilkie, op. cit., 152.
42. M. Ferguson, op. cit., 12–13.
43. W. French Anderson, op. cit., 159.
44. M. Ferguson, op. cit., 14.
45. W. French Anderson, 161.
46 Cited by W. Bodmer and R. McKie, op. cit., 246.
47. *The Lancet.* Cited by W. Bodmer and R. McKie, op. cit., 246.
48. W. French Anderson, 'Uses and abuses of human gene transfer', *Human Gene Therapy* 2 (1992), 1–2.
49. M. de Wachter, 'Ethical Aspects of Human Germ-Line Gene Therapy', *Bioethics* 7 (1993), 167.
50. M. Ferguson, op. cit., 16–19.
51. Ibid., 22–5.
52. J. Harris, *Wonderwoman and Superman*, (Oxford: Oxford University Press, 1992), 44.
53. During the following discussion the embryo's age will be limited to the first 14 days post-fertilisation.
54. H. Leridon, 'Demographie des eches de la reproduction', in *Les Accidents Chromosomiques de la reproduction*. Edited A. Bove and C. Thibault (Paris: Centre International de l'Enfrance, 1973), 13–17.
55. L. Walters, 'Genetics and Reproductive Technologies', in *Medical Ethics*. Edited by R. Veatch (Boston: Jones and Bartlett Publishers, 1989), 204–5.
56. R. Werner, 'Abortion: The Moral Status of the Unborn', *Social Theory and Practice* 3 (1974), 201–2.
57. Ibid., 202.
58. See also R. Wertheimer, 'Understanding the Abortion

Argument', *Philosophy and Public Affairs* 1 (1971): 67–95; B. Brody, 'On the Humanity of the Foetus', in *Contemporary Issues in Bioethics*, edited by T. R. Beauchamp and L. Walter (California: Wadesworth, 1978), 229–40; and T. Iglesias, *IVF and Justice* (London: Linacre Centre for Health Care Ethics, 1990), 97–101.

59. T. Iglesias, 'In Vitro Fertilization: The Major Issues', *Journal of Medical Ethics* 10 (1984), 36.

60. J. Marshall, 'The Case Against Experimentation', in *Experiments on Embryos*, op. cit., 60.

61. N. Ford, *When did I begin?* (Cambridge: Cambridge University Press, 1991), 117.

62. Ibid., 118.

63. Ibid., 119.

64. Ibid., 121.

65. Ibid., 122.

66. J. Harris, *Wonderwoman and Superman* (Oxford: Oxford University Press, 1992), 34–5.

67. G. R. Austin, 'The eggs', in *Germ Cells and Fertilization*, Book 1, *Reproduction in Mammals*. Edited by C. Austin and R. Short, (Cambridge: Cambridge University Press, 1982), 59–61.

68. K. Moore, *The Developing Human: Clinically Oriented Embryology*, 3rd edition (Philadelphia: W. B. Saunders, 1982), 32–3.

69. R. Angell et al, 'Chromosome Abnormalities in Human Embryos after in vitro Fertilization', *Nature* 303 (1983), 336–8.

70. N. Ford, op. cit., 151.

71. K. Dawson, 'Fertilization and Moral Status: A Scientific Perspective', in *Embryo Experimentation*. Edited by P. Singer et al. (Cambridge: Cambridge University Press, 1993), 49.

72. Up to 78% of human fertilisations are lost for a variety of reasons. Refer C. Roberts and C. Lowe, 'Where have all the Conceptions Gone?' *The Lancet* 1 (1975), 498–9.

73. P. Jacobs, 'Pregnancy Losses and Birth Defects', in *Embryonic and Fetal Development: Reproduction in Mammals*, op. cit., 146–7.

74. K. Moore, *The Developing Human: Clinically Oriented Embryology*, 3rd edition (Philadelphia: W. B. Saunders, 1982), 36, 49.

75. B. Ashley and K. O'Rourke, *Health Care Ethics: A Theological Analysis* (St Louis: The Catholic Health Association of the USA, 1982), 223.

76. N. Ford, op. cit., 181.

77. During this process some cells of the epiblast break away and form the mesoblast. This provides some cells to form a layer of intraembryonic mesoderm, while others become the embryonic endoderm, thereby displacing some class from the hypoblast. The cells that are left in the epiblast are now called the embryonic ectoderm. The class of these three layers divide, differentiate, develop and grow into the tissues and organs of the entire embryo proper and fetus. The outer epithelia and the nervous system are derived from the ectoderm. The epithelial linings of the respiratory passages and digestive tract come from the endoderm. The mesoderm gives origin to smooth muscle coats, connective tissues, blood cells, bone marrow, the skeleton and the reproductive and excretory organs. (N. Ford, op. cit., 168).

78 N. Ford, op. cit., 170.

79. A. McLaren, 'Prelude to Embryogenesis', in *Human Embryo Research: Yes or No?* (The CIBA Foundation, London: Tavistock Publications, 1986), 11–12.

80. N. Ford, op. cit., 172.

81. K. Moore, op. cit., 54.

82. A. McLaren, 'Prelude to Embryogenesis', op. cit., 22.

83. N. Ford, op. cit., 175.

84. Ibid., 175.

85. R. Berry, in *The Times*, 6 February 1980 cd 6 15.

86. J. Mahoney, *Bioethics and Beliefs* (London: Sheed and Ward, 1984), 66–7.

87. T. Iglesias, *IVF and Justice* (London: The Linacre Centre for Health Care Ethics, 1990), 97–101.

88. L. Andrews, 'Surrogate Motherhood: The Challenge for Feminists', in *The Ethics of Reproductive Technology*, op. cit., 208.

89. See Rynearson, 'Relinquishment and Its Maternal Complications: A Preliminary Study', *American Journal of Psychiatry* 139 (1982), 338.

90. L. Andrews, op. cit., 209.

91. D. Regan, *NY Testimony* (8 May 1987), Supra Note 10, at 157.

92. L. Andrews, op. cit., 214.

93. Ibid., 217.

94. G. Corea, 'The Mother Machine', in *The Ethics of Reproductive Technology*, op. cit., 225.

95. G. Corea, *The Mother Machine* (London: The Women's Press, 1988), 166–85.

96. Ibid., 3.

97. G. Corea, 'The Mother Machine', op. cit., 228.

98. G. Corea, *The Mother Machine*, op. cit., 7.

99. T. Powledge, 'Unnatural Selection: On Choosing Children's Sex', in *The Custom-made Child? Women-Centered Perspectives*. Edited by H. Holmes et al, (Clifton, NY: Humana Press, 1981), 197.

100. M. Warren, 'The Ethics of Sex Pre-selection', in *The Ethics of Reproductive Technology*, op. cit., 233.

101. M. Baylis, *Reproductive Ethics* (Englewood Cliffs, NJ: Prentice-Hall, 1984), 35.

102. M. Warren, op. cit., 234.

103. B. Adams, 'Birth Order: A Critical Review', *Sociometry* 35 (1972), 411.

104. C. Ernst and J. Angst, *Birth Order: Its Influences on Personality* (Berlin: Springer-Verlag, 1983), 45.

105. D. Kumar, 'Should One be Free to Choose the Sex of One's Child?' in *Ethics, Reproduction and Genetic Control*. Edited by R. Chadwick, (London: Routledge, 1990), 180.

106. M. Warren, op. cit., 244.

107. *Briefing*, 23 November 1984, 6.

108. *Briefing*, 14 December 1984, 3.

109. The Catholic Bishops' Joint Committee on Bio-Ethical Issues on Behalf of the Catholic Bishops of Great Britain, *In Vitro Fertilization: Morality and Public Policy*, Evidence submitted to the Warnock Committee (Catholic Information Services, 1983), no. 25.

110. Ibid., nn. 24 & 26.

111. W. May 'Catholic Moral Teaching on In Vitro Fertilization', in *Reproductive Technologies, Marriage and the Church*. Edited by Pope John Center, (Braintree, Mass: Pope John Center, 1988), 110–12.

112. Congregation for the Doctrine of the Faith, *Instruction on Respect for Human Life in Its origin and on the Dignity of Procreation (Donum Vitae)*, II, B, 4; the internal citation is from Pope Paul VI's *Humanae Vitae*, n. 12.

113. Pope Paul VI, *Humanae Vitae*, 25 July 1968, no. 29. In *Vatican Council II: More Post Conciliar Documents*, Edited by A. Flannery (Dublin: Dominican Publications, 1982), 413.

114. See the New Jersey Catholic Conference on 'Surrogate Motherhood', in *Medical Ethics: Source of Catholic Teaching*. Edited by K. O'Rourke and P. Boyle (St Louis: The Catholic Health Association of the United States of America, 1989), 310.

115. H. Ducharme, 'The Vatican's Dilemma: On the Morality of IVF and the Incarnation', *Bioethics* 5 (1991), 58.

116. Ibid. The internal citation is from Pope Pius XII, 'Discourse to those taking part in the Second Naples World Congress on Fertility and Human Sexuality', 19 May 1956, AAS 48 (1956), 470.

117. *Donum Vitae*, II, B, 4. The internal citation is from the *Code of Canon Law*, c. 1061.

118. P. Ramsey, *Fabricated Man*, (New Haven: Yale University Press, 1970).

119. Refer also, P. Ramsey, '"Shall We Reproduce"? I. The Medical Ethics of in Vitro Fertilization', *JAMA* 220 (1972): 1347; and 'Shall We "Reproduce"? II. Rejoinders and future forecast', *JAMA* 220 (1972): 1480–3.

120. *Donum Vitae*, II, B, 5.

121. *Donum Vitae*, II, B, 5. The internal citation is from Pope John Paul II, *Familiaris Consortio*, n. 14.

122. *Donum Vitae*, II, B, 4, b. The internal citations from Pope John Paul II, 'General Audience on January 16, 1980,' and from Pope John Paul II, 'Discourse on those taking part in the 35th General Assembly of the World Medical Association,' 29 October 1983, AAS 76 (1984), 393.

123. *Catechism of the Catholic Church* (Dublin: Veritas, 1994), no. 2373. Internal quotation is from *Gaudium et Spes*, no. 51.

124. Ibid., n., 2375. Internal quotation taken from *Donum Vitae*, Intro, 2.

125. Ibid., nos 2376 and 2377. Internal quotations from *Donum Vitae* II,1; II,5; II,4.

126. Pope John Paul II, *Evangelium Vitae* (Vatican City: Libreria Editrice Vaticana, 1995), no. 63, 113. See also *Charter of the Rights of the Family* (22 October 1983), article 4b (Vatican Polyglot Press, 1983).

127. Ibid., no. 63, 114.

128. E. Sgreccia, 'Moral Theology and Artificial Procreation in Light of *Donum Vitae*', in *Gift of Life*. Edited by E. Pellegrino, J. Harvey and J. Langan (Washington: Georgetown University Press, 1990), 132–3.

129. *Donum Vitae,* Intro, 5.

130. *Donum Vitae*, Intro, 4.

131. M. Coughlan, *The Vatican, the Law and the Human Embryo* (London: Macmillan, 1990), 76.

132. Congregation for the Doctrine of the Faith, *Declaration on Procured Abortion,* 18 November 1974, footnote 19. Refer A. Flannery, ed., *Vatican Council II: More Post Conciliar Documents,* vol. 2 (Dublin: Dominican Publications, 1982), 552.

133. B. Schuller, 'Paraenesis and Moral Argument in *Donum Vitae*', in *Gift of Love*, op. cit., 81–98.
134. J. Haas, 'The Natural and the Human in Procreation', in *Gift of Love,* op. cit., 97–114.
135. L. Sowle Cahill, 'The Unity of Sex, Love and Procreation', in *Gift of Love*, op. cit., 147.
136. Ibid., 147–8.
137. The Report of a Working Party on Human Fertilization and Embryology of the Board for Social Responsibility, *Personal Origins* (London: CIO Publishing, 1985), n. 106, 38.
138. The Report of a Working Party set up in July 1979 under the auspices of The Free Church Federal Council and the British Council of Churches, *Choices in Childlessness* (1982), 54–5, cf. also 47.
139. Submission to the Warnock Committee prepared by a working party under the auspices of the Baptist Union Department of Mission, and approved by the Baptist Union Council, (March 1983), 8.
140. Board of Social Responsibility: Study Group on Abortion and report on Warnock Report, in *Reports to the General Assembly*, 1985, 290, n. 6.
141. The Methodist Church, *Status of the Unborn Human: As received for discussion and comment by the Methodist Conference 1990*, (Methodist Conference, 1990), 37.
142. *Personal Origins*, n. 99.
143. K. Kelly, *Life and Love* (London: Collins, 1987), 17.
144. *Choices in Childlessness*, op. cit., 42.
145. *Personal Origins*, op. cit., n. 103.
146. Ibid., 37.
147. Ibid., n. 106.
148. K. Kelly, op. cit., 19.
149. Ibid., 46.
150. Board of Social Responsibility: Study Group on Abortion and Report on Warnock Report, in *Reports to the General Assembly*, 1985, 290.
151. Ibid., 289.
152. *Human Fertilization and Embryology*, The Response of the Board for Social Responsibility of the General Synod of the Church of England to the DHSS Report of the Committee of Enquiry (1984), n. 5.2.
153. *Personal Origins*, n. 108.
154. *Personal Origins*, n. 109.
155. Ibid., n. 107.

156. Ibid., n. 110.
157. Ibid., n. 113.
158. Ibid., n. 112.
159. Board for Social Responsibility, *Legislation on Human Infertility Services and Embryo Research* (London: General Synod of the Church of England, 1988), n. 5.
160. *Legislation on Human Infertility Services and Embryo Research*, n. 6.
161. *Personal Origins*, n. 133.
162. Ibid., n. 134.
163. Ibid., n. 135.
164. Ibid., n. 137.
165. Ibid., n. 138.
166. *Legislation on Human Infertility Services and Embryo Research*, n. 7.
167. 'Bishop opposes abortion but supports treatment', *The Independent*, 8 January 1994, 2.
168. Ibid., 2.
169. Submission to the Warnock Committee prepared by a working party under the auspices of the Baptist Union Department of Mission, and approved by the Baptist Union Council (March 1983), n. 13.
170. Ibid., n. 13.
171. Ibid., n. 13.
172. Ibid., n. 13.
173. Ibid., n. 14.
174. Ibid., n. 15.
175. The Methodist Church, *The Status of the Unborn Human: As received for discussion and comment by the Methodist Conference 1990*, (London: Methodist Publishing House, 1990), n. 6.2.3.
176. Ibid., n. 6.3.1.
177. Ibid., n 6.3.2.
178. Ibid., n 6.3.2.
179. Ibid., n. 6.3.3.
180. Ibid., n. 6.6.3.
181. K. Kelly, op. cit., 35–6.

Chapter 3 (pages 123–177)
  1. *The Independent*, 8 January 1994, 14.
  2. The survey of 12,800 people was carried out in 1993 to gauge public acceptance of bio-technology and human genetic treatments.

3. T. Wilkie, 'Society agonizes in the race to keep up with laboratory', *The Independent*, 8 January 1994, 6.
4. D. J. Weatherall, 'The New Genetics', in *New Prospects for Medicine*. Edited by J. Austyn (Oxford: Oxford University Press, 1988), 43.
5. Nuffield Council on Bioethics, *Genetic Screening: Ethics Issues* (London: Nuffield Council on Bioethics, 1993), 7.
6. D. Weatherall, op. cit., 46–7.
7. P. Elmer-Dewitt, 'The Genetic Revolution', *Time*, 17 January 1994, 35.
8. LeRoy Walters, 'Genetics and Reproductive Technologies', in *Medical Ethics*. Edited by R. Veatch (Boston: Jones and Bartlett Publishers, 1989), 215–16.
9. Huntington's disease is an inherited disorder affecting about one person in every 10,000 in the UK. The abnormal gene was isolated as recently as March 1993. It is a progressive disease of the central nervous system, characterised by involuntary movements, loss of motor control and dementia. The symptoms most commonly first appear in individuals of between 40 and 50 years of age, with death occurring 15–20 years later.
10. Down's syndrome is a genetic disorder, but not inherited, it affects about 1 in 600 babies born overall, although the risk of having a child with Down's syndrome rises sharply when the mother is over 35 years of age. The vast majority of individuals with Down's syndrome have an extra copy of chromosome 21, are born with specific physical characteristics and have severe learning disabilities. A very small percentage are inherited due to a translocation.
11. Refer Nuffield Council on Bioethics, op. cit., 8–9.
12. Cystic fibrosis (CF) is a serious inherited disease affecting the lungs and digestive system of babies, children and young adults. People with CF have sticky mucus in their lungs and are particularly prone to chest infections. They also have difficulty in digesting foods, especially fatty foods, and may later develop liver problems. Treatment (antibiotics, physiotherapy, digestive enzymes) can greatly help but does not cure the condition. The average life expectancy of a person with CF is about 20 to 30 years. The disorder is inherited and the change in the gene responsible for about 85% of the cases can now be detected. For the disease to develop, a defective gene must be inherited from each parent. Parents who have only one of a pair of defective genes are known as carriers and are themselves completely healthy. About 1 in 20 of the white population in the UK are

carriers of the gene; the disease occurs in about 1 in 2,000 babies born. If both parents are carriers, the risk of any baby having the disease is 1 in 4.

13. Haemophilia is a descriptive name of a group of blood disorders, all of which have clotting problems as the basic defect. The most common type, haemophilia A, affects about 1 in 10,000 live male births. Individuals affected with haemophilia A are unable to produce normal factor VIII, one of a number of factors associated with the clotting mechanism of the blood. Manifestations of the disease include haemorrhages in joints following only minimal injury, bruising in soft tissues from minor bumps, and severe bleeding from minor injuries. Arthritis is a frequent complication. Bleeding episodes can be limited by the prompt infusion of factor VIII, but use of contaminated preparations in the early 1980s caused infection of many haemophiliacs with human immunodeficiency virus (HIV).

14. Familial hypercholesterolaemia: High levels of blood cholesterol are associated with an increased risk of heart disease, especially in men in middle age. In most individuals, raised blood cholesterol results from the interaction of several genes (not all of which have been identified) and environmental factors, such as a high fat diet.

Familial hypercholesterolaemia is the name given to a specific inherited disorder in which the gene causes high levels of blood cholesterol from birth. It is dominantly inherited and individuals with a single abnormal gene have a greatly increased risk of developing heart disease by the age of 50 years; those who inherit the abnormal gene from both parents have extremely high blood cholesterol and many develop heart disease in their teens. It is estimated that about 1 in 500 individuals are born with the disorder but the very serious (both genes affected) condition only occurs in about 1 in 1,000,000.

15. Breast cancer: It is believed that several genes play a role in the 25,000 new cases of breast cancer diagnosed in Britain every year, particularly where onset is early or where multiple family members are affected. A gene that predisposes women in some families to breast cancer has been traced to a region of chromosome 17 and it is likely that the gene itself will soon be isolated.

Familial colorectal cancer: Colorectal cancer causes about 20,000 deaths each year in Britain and yet if diagnosed at an early stage it is curable. Two relatively common types of inherited predisposition to cancer of the colon have been identified.

Familial adenomatous polyposis is a dominantly inherited disease accounting for about 1% of colon cancer patients and has a birth frequency of about 1 in 8,000. Individuals with the disorder develop hundred of polyps in the colon during adolescence, and typically develop colorectal cancer by the fourth decade. The gene responsible has been identified, making it possible to offer genetic testing to individuals at risk, and to provide prophylactic treatment (surgery to remove the colon) to individuals found to be affected.

Hereditary non-polyposis colon cancer may cause between 5% and 15% of cases of colorectal cancer. Individuals with the abnormal gene do not develop numerous polyps, but those that do occur rapidly become cancerous. This form of colon cancer is thought to be associated with a gene on chromosome 2, but other genes may also be involved.

16. Turner's syndrome affects girls who have only one normal X chromosome instead of the usual complement of two. It occurs in about 1 in 50,000 girls and is usually not inherited. Over 99% of girls with Turner's syndrome are infertile, due to lack of fully developed ovaries. The most obvious feature in childhood is short stature; there may also be heart defects. Intelligence is generally normal, but there may be some learning difficulties.

17. Nuffield Council of Bioethics, op. cit., 10.

18. Sickle Cell Disease: an inherited abnormality of haemoglobin (called haemoglobin S) in the red blood cells may cause deformity of the cells known as sickling. Those at most risk of inheriting sickle cell disorders are people of African, African/Asian Caribbean, Eastern Mediterranean, Asian and Middle Eastern origin. The inheritance of one sickle cell gene generally causes no problems; individuals who inherit the gene from each parent have sickle cell disease.

A child born with sickle cell disease does not generally have problems until after the age of four to six months. After this age most children become anaemic because the sickle cells are destroyed in the blood. The children may also from time to time get additional problems such as hard foot syndrome (swelling of the hands and feet), mild to excruciating pains throughout the body, chest infections, strokes and damage to various parts of the body including the hips, shoulders, eyes and lungs. These are due to the sickle cells causing blockage of smaller blood vessels and other problems. The majority of affected individuals survive into adulthood but there are occasional deaths of young children and adults due to complications such as overwhelming infections and sickling in the spleen and lungs.

19. Thalassaemia is the name given to a group of inherited disorders of haemoglobin production and can be broadly divided into two types: alpha thalassaemia and beta thalassaemia, both of which are recessively inherited.

Most people with alpha thalassaemia originate from the Far East, notably Hong Kong, China, Singapore and Vietnam; as well as from Cyprus, Greece and the Middle East. There are two types of alpha thalassaemia, but generally only the severe type is clinically important. It causes a total absence of haemoglobin production in the fetus, leading to stillbirth, usually before the expected date of delivery.

The main groups at risk of inheriting beta thalassaemia are people of Mediterranean and Southern European, Asian and Middle Eastern and Far Eastern origin. A child with this form of thalassaemia is unable to make a sufficient amount of haemoglobin and will develop anaemia in early childhood if not treated with frequent blood transfusions. However, this treatment causes too much iron to be stored in the body, so the child has to be taught to use an infusion pump to get rid of this excess iron and this is a burdensome procedure. Since the advent of treatment early in life, children are now surviving into their twenties or thirties, and more recently bone marrow transplantation has further improved the prognosis.

20. Enlarged kidneys with cysts.
21. Heart muscle disease.
22. Nuffield Council on Bioethics, 10–13.
23. Rhesus haemolytic disease can occur if the mother's blood group is rhesus negative and the father's is rhesus positive (about 85% of people are rhesus positive and 15% are rhesus negative). In this situation, the fetus may also be rhesus positive. If sufficient leakage of fetal blood into the maternal circulation occurs, which is particularly likely at the time of delivery, a rhesus negative woman can develop antibodies against the rhesus positive blood group and subsequent babies may be affected, with destruction of their blood cells causing anaemia and jaundice. Very severely affected infants have problems before birth; after birth treatment (exchange transfusion) may be needed to correct anaemia and prevent brain damage due to jaundice.

The condition used to cause 1–2 per 1,000 stillbirths or deaths in the newborn period. It is now largely prevented by screening all pregnant women for their rhesus blood group early in pregnancy and ensuring that all are given an injection of antibody within a few hours of delivery (or miscarriage). This removes any fetal rhesus positive cells from the mother's bloodstream and so prevents her becoming immunised in almost every case.

24. PKU is a rare inherited disorder, affecting about 1 in 10,000 births in the UK. Affected individuals inherit the abnormal gene from each parent and are unaffected at birth; but with the introduction of feeding a substance in the blood builds up and causes brain damage, so that untreated children become severely mentally handicapped. Every baby in the UK has a blood test for PKU at about six days of age and if the diagnosis is confirmed, a special diet is started. With rigorous dietary control mental development can be normal, although the intellectual status of early treated subjects is not as good as was originally thought. The dietary control has to be continued at least into late childhood and possibly throughout life. Women with PKU require particularly strict dietary control during pregnancy. The current screening test only detects babies who may be affected.

25. Severe learning difficulty due to fragile X syndrome distinguished by a visible change near the tip of the X chromosome, is thought to occur in approximately one in every 2,000 male births. The mode of transmission is complicated, because the change in the gene tends to increase with successive generations, and some males can be unaffected, yet transmit the carrier state to their daughters. Girls may also be affected, but to a lesser degree: about one-third of girls carrying this genetic abnormality will have some degree of learning difficulty.

Severe learning difficulty is the main characteristic of the disorder, although this varies markedly in severity between individuals. There is no limitation of life expectancy for children with fragile X syndrome.

26. Nuffield Council on Bioethics, op. cit., 15–17.
27. J. Wilson and G. Junger, *Principles and Practice of Screening for Disease*, Public Health Papers WHO no. 34, (Geneva: WHO, 1968). As cited in D. Macer, *Shaping Genes* (Christchurch, New Zealand: Eubios Ethics Institute, 1990), 240.
28. M. Lappe, J. Gustafson and R. Roblin, 'Ethical and Social Issues in Screening for Genetic Disease', *The New England Journal of Medicine* vol. 286:21 (1972), 1129–32.
29. Committee on the Ethics of Gene Therapy, *Report of the Committee on the Ethics of Gene Therapy* (London: HMSO, 1992).
30. Nuffield Council on Bioethics, op. cit., 17–18.
31. Congenital hypothyroidism: abnormal development or function

of the thyroid gland resulting in lack of production of thyroid hormone occurs in about one in 4,000 babies in the UK. The baby is usually normal at birth because the mother's thyroxine has been able to pass to the baby. Unless treatment with thyroxine is started within the first few weeks of life, growth and mental development will be delayed. Screening is carried out by measuring specific hormones in the blood taken from the baby at around the end of the first week.

32. Duchenne's muscular dystrophy (DMD) is a serious progressive disease of muscles affecting about one in 3,500 newborn boys. There are no signs of disease at birth, and affected boys develop and grow normally until around 18 months of age. From the ages of 7 to 12, affected boys become wheelchair bound. Death from chest infection or heart failure usually occurs by the early 20s or before.

   About a third of cases arise from new mutations and are not inherited from carrier mothers. Women carrying the abnormal gene have a 1 in 2 risk of having a son with the disorder; 1 in 2 of their daughters will be carriers.

33. D. Bradley, E. Parsons, and E. Clark, 'Experience with screening newborns for Duchenne's muscular dystrophy in Wales', *British Medical Journal* 306 (1993), 357–60.

34. S. Zeesman, C. Clow, L. Cartier and C. Scriver, 'A private view of heterozygosity: eight year follow-up study on carriers of the Tay-Sachs gene detected by high school screening in Montreal', *American Journal of Human Genetics* 36 (1984), 769–78.

35. Amniocentesis: The most widely used technique of pre-natal diagnosis, most commonly carried out at 15–18 weeks gestation, although it can be carried out as early as 12 weeks. Ultrasound is used to locate the placenta, and a small quantity of amniotic fluid, which contains cells shed by the developing fetus, is withdrawn through a needle from the amniotic cavity. Cells have to be cultured before chromosome examination (for example, to detect Down's syndrome) or DNA analysis can take place. Genetic diagnosis is not usually possible until 16–20 weeks of pregnancy. There is still some uncertainty about the exact risk to the pregnancy from amniocentesis largely because the risk is so low that it is extremely difficult to measure. The best studies suggest a 0.5–1% excess risk of spontaneous abortion following amniocentesis at 15–16 weeks and a slightly increased incidence of mild respiratory problems in the newborn. Good data are not yet available on the risks of early amniocentesis.

36. Chorionic villus sampling (CVS) is a procedure whereby a small

sample of chorionic (placental) tissue, which shares the genetic make up of the fetus, is removed for pre-natal diagnosis. It is usually performed at about 10 weeks of pregnancy with only minimal discomfort and often allows a genetic diagnosis to be achieved before 12 weeks' gestation. CVS requires first-class ultrasound and an expert and well-trained team. The risks are higher than for amniocentesis: an MRC trial gave 2–4% excess miscarriage risk.

37. If rubella (German measles) is contracted in the early stages of pregnancy (before about 12 weeks) it can cause stillbirths or serious congenital malformations such as blindness, deafness, heart defects and mental retardation. As a result of programmes both for immunising schoolgirls and non-pregnant women against the virus, and by screening during pregnancy, the incidence of children born with severe congenital rubella syndromes has declined from about 3.5 to 0.41 per 100,000 births between 1980 and 1985 in most of Western Europe.

38. Neural Tube Defects: These conditions occur if the brain and/or the spinal cord with its protecting skull and spinal column fail to develop properly. They include anencephaly, where most of the brain and skull are absent and stillbirth or death soon after delivery is inevitable, and spina bifida, where the spinal canal is not enclosed and the spinal cord and nerves may be damaged. Infants born with spina bifida show a wide range of physical disabilities and in the most severe forms the legs and bladder may be paralysed. The causes of NTD are complex, but there is an undoubted genetic component, the risk for subsequent offspring after the birth of an affected child being increased about tenfold.

39. Nuffield Council on Bioethics, op. cit., 18–26.

40. B. Modell. Cited by W. Bodmer and R. McKie, *The Book of Man: The Quest to Discover Our Genetic Heritage* (London: Little, Brown and Company, 1994), 234.

41. Ibid., 234.

42. Ibid., 234–46.

43. N. Scarisbrick. Cited in W. Bodmer and R. McKie, op. cit., 236.

44. W. Bodmer and R. McKie, op. cit., 236.

45. P. Rowley. Cited by W. Bodmer and R. McKie, op. cit., 238.

46. W. Bodmer and M. Bodmer, op. cit., 238–9.

47. Ibid., 240–41.

48. W. French Anderson, 'Genetics and human malleability', *Hastings Center Report* 20 (1990), 21–24.

49. T. T. Juengst, 'Germ-line gene therapy: back to basics,' *Journal of Medicine and Philosophy* 16 (1991), 589–90.

50. M. Warnock, cited by T. Wilkie, op. cit., 159.
51. J. Harris, *Wonderwoman and Superman* (Oxford: Oxford University Press, 1992), 201–2.
52. M. Warnock. Cited by T. Wilkie, op. cit., 162.
53. Ibid.
54. T. Wilkie, op. cit., 165.
55. Report of the Committee on the Ethics of Gene Therapy, London, HMSO, 1992 (Clothier Report), 9.
56. R. M. Cook-Deegan, 'Human gene therapy and Congress', *Human Gene Therapy* 1 (1990), 163–70.
57. R. Wimmer, '"Kategorische Argumente" gegen die Keimbahn-Gentherapie', in *Ethik ohne Chance?* Edited by J. Wils and D. Mieth, (Tubingen, 1991), 182–209.
58. European Medical Research Councils, 'Gene therapy in man', *The Lancet*, 1988, 1271–2.
59. Comite Consultatif National de'Ethique, 'Avis sur la therapie genique. Paris 1991', *Human Gene Therapy* 2 (1991), 329.
60. Department of Health, NHS Management Executive, undated, Chapter 1, paragraph 2.
61. Nuffield Council on Bioethics, op. cit., 30–31.
62. LeRoy Walters, 'Genetics and Reproductive Technologies', op. cit., 216–17.
63. W. Bodmer and R. McKie, op. cit., 242.
64. Nuffield Council on Bioethics, op. cit., 42–3.
65. Report of the Committee on Privacy, Cmnd 5012 (1972), 10.
66. Nuffield Council on Bioethics, op. cit., 44–5.
67. Ibid., 45.
68. J. Haldane, *Heredity and Politics* (London: Allen and Unwin, 1938), 179, as cited by T. H. Murray, 'The Human Genome Project and Genetic Testing: Ethical Implications', in *The Genome, Ethics and the Law* (Washington, DC: American Association for the Advancement of Science, 1992), 62.
69. T. Murray, op. cit., 63.
70. Nuffield Council on Bioethics, op. cit., 56.
71. Ibid., 56–7.
72. Ibid., 61.
73. Ibid., 62.
74. S. Gevers, 'Use of Genetic Data, Employment and Insurance: An International Perspective', *Bioethics* 7 (1993), 128.
75. G. Atherley, 'Human Rights versus Occupational Medicine', *International Journal of Health Services* 13 (1983), 265–75.
76. T. Murray, 'Ethical Issues in Human Genome Research', *FASEB Journal* 5 (1991), 57.

77. International Labour Organisation, *Occupational Health Services Recommendation* (Geneva), 1985.
78. Health Council of the Netherlands, *Heredity: Science and Society* (The Hague, 1989).
79. European Parliament, Resolution on the Ethical and Legal Problems of Genetic Engineering, *Official Journal of the European Commission*, 17 April 1989, no. C69, 165–73.
80. R. Fisher, *Linkage studies and the prognosis of hereditary aliments* (London: International Congress on Life Assurance Medicine, 1935), 1–3.
81. Nuffield Council on Bioethics, op. cit., 65.
82. Ibid., 66.
83. See Art 12 of the UN International Covenant on Economic, Social and Cultural Rights.
84. H. Roscam Abbing, 'Genetic Predictive Testing and Private Insurance', *Health Policy* 18 (1991), 197–206.
85. See on actuarial fairness as opposed to moral fairness: N. Daniels, 'Insurability and the HIV Epidemic: Ethical Issues in Underwriting', *Milbank Quarterly* 68 (1990), 497–525.
86. Nuffield Council on Bioethics, op. cit., 67.
87. S. Gevers, op. cit., 130.
88. Council of Europe, *Recommendation on Genetic Testing and Screening for Health Care Purposes* no. R (92) 3, Strasbourg, 1992.
89. S. Gevers, op. cit., 131.
90. Abschlussbericht der Bund-Lander-Arbeitsgruppe Genomanalyse, Bundesanzeiger 1990; 42, no. 161a, 44–6.
91. 'Proposed Ban on Genetic Testing in Denmark', *The Lancet* 337 (1991), 1340.
92. A comparable suggestion has been made in *Recommendation 1116 (1989) on AIDS and Human Rights* of the Parliamentary Assembly of the Council of Europe.
93. G. Atkinson and A. Moraczewski, *Genetic Counselling, the Church and the Law: A Report of The Task Force on Genetic Diagnosis and Counselling* (St Louis, Missouri: Pope John XXIII Medical-Moral Research and Education Center, 1980), 143–4.
94. K. Rahner, 'The Problem of Genetic Manipulation', in *Theological Investigations*, vol. 9 (New York: Herder and Herder, 1972). A sympathetic exposition of Rahner's ideas are given by the catholic moral theologian Bernard Häring in *Ethics and Manipulation* (New York: Seabury Press, 1975).
95. J. Nelson, *On the New Frontiers of Genetics and Religion* (Grand Rapids, Michigan: Eerdmans, 1994), 15–16.

96. Pope John Paul II, Discourse to students at Cologne, 15 November 1980, cited in Discourse to the Pontifical Academy of Sciences, 28 October 1986, AAS 79 (1987), 873.

97. For example, Pope John XXIII's *Pacem in terris*, and Paul VI's *Humanae Vitae*, nn 4, 12.

98. B. Johnstone, 'The Human Genome Project: Catholic Theological Perspective', in *The Interaction of Catholic Bioethics and Secular Society: Proceedings of the Eleventh Bishops' Workshop Dallas, Texas*. Edited by R. Smith (Braintree, Massachusetts: Pope John XXIII Center, 1992), 268.

99. J. Monod, *Chance and Necessity* (London: Collins, 1972). E. O. Wilson, *Sociobiology: The New Synthesis* (Cambridge, Mass: Harvard University Press, 1975). E. O. Wilson, *On Human Nature* (Cambridge, Mass: Harvard University Press, 1978).

100. H. Jonas, *The Imperative of Responsibility: In Search of an Ethics for the Technological Age* (Chicago: The University of Chicago Press, 1984), 205.

101. B. Johnstone, op. cit., 268–9.

102. John Paul II, To those gathered for the convention of biological experimentation in Vatican City, 23 October 1982, AAS 75 (1983), 35–9.

103. B. Johnstone, op. cit., 269.

104. Ibid., 270.

105. John Paul II, *Centesimus Annus*, no. 37.

106. K. Demmer, 'Natur und Person: Brennpunkte gegenwartige moraltheologischer Auseinandersetzung', in *Natur im ethischen Argument,* ed., B. Fraling (Freiburg: Universitatsverlag, 1990), 55–86.

107. J. Reiter, 'Pradiktive Medizin–Genomanalyse–Gentherapie', *Internationale katholische Zeitschrift* (Communio) 19 (1990), 120.

108. *The Catechism of the Universal Church* (Dublin: Veritas, 1994), no. 2274, 490. Refer *Donum Vitae*, I, 2.

109. *Catechism*, op. cit., no. 2275, 490. Refer *Donum Vitae*, I, 6.

110. Pope John Paul II, *Evangelium Vitae* (Vatican City: Libreria Editrice Vaticana, 1995), no. 63, 114.

111. B. Johnstone, op. cit., 271.

112. When asked by John's disciples, 'Are you, "He who is to come" or do we look for another?' Jesus responded with words recalling the prophecies of Isaiah: 'Go back and report to John what you hear and see; the blind recover their sight, cripples walk, lepers are cured, the deaf hear, dead men are raised to life, and the poor have the good news preached to them' (Mt. 11:3–5).

113. "'Which is less trouble to say, 'Your sins are forgiven' or 'Stand up and walk?' To help you realise that the Son has authority on earth to forgive sins". He then said to the paralysed man: "Stand up! Roll up your mat and go home."' (Mt. 9:5f).

114. National Conference of Catholic Bishops, *Pastoral Statement of U.S. Catholic Bishops on Handicapped People* (Washington, DC: United States Catholic Conference, 1978), 2.

115. Ibid., 3.

116. G. Atkinson and A. Moraczewski, op. cit., 146.

117. H. Jonas, *The Imperative of Responsibility: In Search of an Ethics for the Technological Age* (Chicago: Chicago University Press, 1984), 203.

118. F. Boeckle, 'General Ethics of Genome Manipulation', in *The International Conference on Bioethics: The Human Genome Sequencing: Ethical Issues*, Tome 10–15 April 1989 (Brescia: CLAS International, 1989), 252.

119. Cf. E. Shelp, ed., *Virtue and Medicine: Explorations in the Character of Medicine* (Dordrecht: D. Reidal, 1985).

120. B. Johnstone, op. cit., 273.

121. Ibid., 274.

122. R. McCormick, 'Genetic Technology and Our Common Future' in *The Critical Call: Reflections on Moral Dilemmas Since Vatican II* (Washington, DC: Georgetown University Press, 1989), 270.

123. *Instruction on Respect for Human Life in its Origin and on the Dignity of Procreation (Donum Vitae)*, (Vatican City: Libreria Editrice Vaticana, 1987), Introduction, no. 3.

124. John Paul II, 'The Ethics of Genetic Manipulation', *Origins* 13 (1983): 385–9. A more recent statement, but without further specification of detailed norms can be found in John Paul II, Discourse to The Pontifical Academy of Sciences, 28 October 1986, AAS 79 (1987), 878. This quote is taken from an earlier address on the same subject, 23 October 1982, AAS 75 (1983), 37–8.

125. John Paul II, 'The Ethics', 388.

126. B. Johnstone, op. cit., 275–6.

127. F. Boeckle, 'General Ethics', op. cit., 260.

128. P. Ramsey, 'Shall we "Reproduce"?', *Journal of the American Medical Association* 220 (5 June 1972), 1347.

129. Ibid., 1480f.

130. J. Fletcher, 'Ethical aspects of genetic controls: designed genetic changes in man', *New England Journal of Medicine* 285 (1971), 779.

131. Ibid., 780.
132. *Faith and Science in an Unjust World*, ed. P. Abrecht, vol. 2 (Geneva: World Council of Churches, 1980), 49.
133. Ibid., 54.
134. *Experiments with Man: report of an Ecumenical Consultation*, edited by Hans-Ruedi Weber (New York: World Council of Churches and Friendship Press, 1969), 13.
135. A. Dyson, 'Genetic Engineering in Theology', in *Ethics and Biotechnology*. Edited by A. Dyson and J. Harris (London: Routledge, 1994), 262.
136. Report of a Working Party on Human Fertilization and Embryology of the Board for Social Responsibility, *Personal Origins* (London: CIO Publishers, 1985), 18–19.
137. Ibid., 12.
138. *Manipulating Life: Ethical Issues in Genetic Engineering* (Geneva: World Council of Churches, 1982).
139. Ibid., 3.
140. Ibid., 5.
141. Ibid., 7.
142. Ibid., 8.
143. Ibid., 11.
144. *Biotechnology: The Challenge to the Churches and to the World* (Geneva: World Council of Churches, August 1989).
145. J. Nelson, op. cit., 172–5.

Chapter 4 (pages 178–247)
1. C. Koop, 'The Right to Die: The Moral Dilemmas', in *Euthanasia: The Moral Issues*. Edited by R. Baird and S. Rosenbaum (New York: Prometheus Books, 1989), 69.
2. M. Kohl, 'Beneficent Euthanasia', *The Humanist* 34 (July/August 1974), 9.
3. R. Gillon, 'Suicide and Voluntary Euthanasia: Historical Perspective', in *Euthanasia and the Right to Death*. Edited by A. B. Downing (Los Angeles: Nash Publishing, 1969), 173–92.
4. Seneca, *Laws* IX:843.
5. R. Wennberg, *Terminal Choices* (Grand Rapids, Michigan: William B. Eerdmans, 1989), 2.
6. L. Weatherhead, *The Christian Agnostic* (New York: Abingdon Press, 1965), 269.
7. H. Rashdall, *The Theory of Good and Evil*, 2nd ed. (Oxford: Oxford University Press, 1924), 209.
8. W. Inge, *Christian Ethics and Modern Problems* (New York: G. P. Putnam's Sons, 1930), 393–8.

9. J. Wilson, *Death by Decision* (Philadelphia: Westminster Press, 1975).

10. J. Fletcher, *Morals and Medicine* (Boston: Beacon Press, 1954), 172–210.

11. C. Curran, *Politics, Medicine, and Christian Ethics: A Dialogue with Paul Ramsey* (Philadelphia: Fortress Press, 1973), 152–63.

12. D. Maguire, *Death by Choice* (New York: Schocken Books, 1975).

13. J. Sullivan, 'The Immorality of Euthanasia', in *Beneficent Euthanasia*. Edited M. Kohl (Buffalo, NY: Prometheus Books, 1975), 19.

14. R. Wennberg, op. cit., 3.

15. E. Noelle-Neumann and E. Piel (eds.), *Allensbacher Jahrbuch der Demoskopie* 1978–83, vol. 8 (Muhchen, 1983), 172; quoted in *Euthanasie oder soll man auf Verlangen toten?* Edited by V. Eid (Mainz: Matthias-Grunewald, 1985), 188ff.

16. For the first two figures see W. Monahan, 'Contemporary American Opinion on Euthanasia', in *Moral Responsibility in Prolonging Life Decisions*. Edited by D. McCarthy and A. Moraczewski (St Louis, Mo: Pope John Center, 1981), 181; for the last figure see Newsweek, 18 June 1990, 37.

17. *Newsweek*, 14 March 1988, 46.

18. M. Kidron and R. Segal, *The New State of the World Atlas* (London: Simon & Schuster, 1991), 37.

19. P. van der Mass, J. van Delden, L. Pijnenborg and C. Looman, 'Euthanasia and Other Medical Decisions Concerning the End of Life', *The Lancet*, 14 September 1991, cited in *The Tablet*, 19 October 1991, 1293 and 1294.

20. Pope John Paul II, *Evangelium Vitae* (Vatican City: Libreria Editrice Vaticana, 1995), nos 69–70.

21. Individuals are likely to take into consideration not only suffering in the sense of an adverse appreciation of pain, but also the psychological and social costs that their further life will likely impose on those for whom they care and on society generally. The costly prolongation of life may expend family resources, which the individual would rather have invested in other undertakings (e.g. sending children to college). Finally, the person may find continued existence under certain circumstances to be undignified and unacceptable from an aesthetic point of view.

22. Cf. R. Gula, *What Are They Saying About Euthanasia?* (New York/Mahwah: Paulist Press, 1986), 104.

23. 'Let us note that most of the time the physician tends to

minimize if not even deny the burden of the physical and moral sufferings of the patient being subjected to a reanimation. The noise, the illumination, the lack of sleep, the continuous making of probes, the extraordinary dependence of the one whose respiration, nutrition, depuration depend on artificial means, arms and legs often immobilised, the agitation of the personnel around the other patients and, at the end of all this, the not indifferent risk of a survival burdened by heavy handicaps, all that scenography goes at the expense of the patient.' P. Verspieren, *Eutanasia? Dall'accanimento terapeutico all'accompagnamento dei morenti* (Torino: Ed. Paoline, 1985), 26.

24. H. Saner, in *Malattia, eutanasia, morte nella discussione contemporanea*. Edited by A. Bondolfi (Bologna: EDB, 1989), 143. 'Under the aegis of treatment, he (the patient) is being tortured with a cruelty which nature would not be capable of' (128).

25. J. Wunderli, 'Probleme am Lebensende', in *Medizin im Widerspruch*. Edited by J. Wunderli and K. Weishaupt (Olten, 1977), 213; quoted by F. Furger and K. Koch, *Verfugbares Leben?* (Freiburg/Schweiz: Nationalkommission Justitia et Pax, 1978), 62.

26. 'Under the pretext to respect life, the physicians arrogate to themselves the right to inflict upon human beings any torture and every humiliation. This is called doing their duty', P. Verspieren, op. cit., 23.

27. H. Engelhardt, 'Death by Free Choice', in *Suicide and Euthanasia*. Edited by B. Brody (London: Kluwer Academic Publishers, 1989), 253–5.

28. S. Wanzer, et al, 'The Physician's Responsibility toward Hopelessly Ill Patients: A Second Look', *The New England Journal of Medicine* 320 (13), (30 March 1989), 844–9.

29. J. Drane, *Clinical Bioethics* (Kansas City: Sheed and Ward, 1994), 87.

30. K. Kearon, 'New Law, New Twist to Euthanasia Debate', *The Irish Times*, 21 February 1995, 14.

31. *Time*, 12 June 1995, 37.

32. J. Kevorkian, *Prescription: Medicide* (Buffalo, NY, 1991). Kevorkian gives a good account of his own actions.

33. For details of the Zygmaniak case, see P. Mitchell, *Act of Love* (New York, 1976), or the *New York Times*, 1, 3, and 6 November 1973.

34. P. Singer, *Practical Ethics*, 2nd edition (Cambridge: Cambridge University Press, 1993), 178.

35. An 'Advance Directive' or 'Living Will' is an instruction that one wishes to have treatment withdrawn or withheld in specific circumstances (i.e. when one is unconscious/in pain/no longer able to give consent etc.). In *Bland* the English Law Lords appear to have ruled that 'Advanced Directives' or 'Living Wills' were legal documents, and should be respected as such.

36. R. Campbell and D. Collinson, *Ending Lives* (Oxford: Basil Blackwell, 1991), 123.

37. Louis Repouille's killing of his son was reported in the *New York Times*, 13 October 1939, and is cited by Yale Kamisar, 'Some Non-religious Views against Proposed Mercy Killing Legislation', *Minnesota Law Review*, vol. 42 (1958), 1,021.

38. Details of the Linares case are from the *New York Times*, 27 April 1989 and the *Hastings Center Report,* July/August 1989.

39. P. Singer, op. cit., 176–81.

40. E. Bartlett and S. Youngner, 'Human Death and the Destruction of the Neocortex', in *Death: Beyond Whole-Brain Criteria.* Edited R. Zaner (Dordrecht: Kluwer Academic Publishers, 1988), 200.

41. D. Brock, *Life and Death* (Cambridge: Cambridge University Press, 1993), 145.

42. C. Culver and B. Gert, *Philosophy in Medicine: Conceptual and Ethical Dilemmas in Medicine and Psychiatry* (New York: Oxford University Press, 1982).

43. Law reform Commission of Canada, *Report on the Criteria for the Determination of Death* (Ottawa: Ministry of Supply and Service, 1981).

44. The President's Commission for the study of Ethical Problems in Medicine and Biomedical and Behaviourial Research, *Defining Death: Medical, Legal and Ethical Issues in the Determination of Death* (Washington DC: US Government Printing Office, 1981).

45. B. A. Rix, 'Danish Ethics Council Rejects Brain Death as the Criterion for Death', *Journal of Medical Ethics* 16 (1990), 5–7.

46. President's Commission for Ethical Problems in Medicine, *Defining Death* (Washington DC: Government Printing Office, 1981), 38.

47. C. Culver and B. Gert, op. cit., 180.

48. C. Pallis, *ABC of Brainstem Death* (London: British Medical Association, 1983); C. Pallis, 'Death', in *Encyclopedia Britannica*, 1986.

49. D. Lamb, *Death, Brain Death and Ethics* (London: Croom Helm, 1988).

50. C. Pallis, op. cit., 10–21.
51. M. Evans, 'Against the definition of brainstem death', in *Death Rites*. Edited by R. Lee and D. Morgan (London: Routledge, 1994), 1.
52. This phrase is not used by Pallis himself; it is offered by David Lamb, *Death, Brain Death and Ethics* (London: Croom Helm, 1985), and it serves as a useful shorthand for the notion which Pallis does employ: the role of an organ whose loss implies the death of some larger organ as a whole or, in the ultimate case, of the human being as a whole.
53. C. Pallis, op. cit., 1–8.
54. C. Pallis, op. cit., 30.
55. Pallis refers to a Danish study which showed that the maximum heart functioning was 72–211 hours.
56. See M. Evans and D. Hill, 'The brainstems of organ donors are not dead', *Catholic Medical Quarterly* XL 3 (243) (August 1989), 9, for a detailed and authoritatively referenced discussion of persistent brainstem functions.
57. M. Green and D. Wikler, 'Brain Death and Personal Identity', *Philosophy and Public Affairs* 9 (1980), 105–33; R. Veatch, 'The Whole-Brain Oriented Concept of Death: An Outmoded Philosophical Formulation', *Journal of Thanatology* 13 (1975).
58. D. Brock, *Life and Death*, op. cit., 146–7.
59. J. Harris, *The Value of Life* (London: Routledge & Kegan Paul, 1985), 8–9.
60. J. Harris, op. cit., 241–2.
61. J. Fletcher, *Humanhood: Essays in Biomedical Ethics* (Buffalo: Prometheus Books, 1979), 7–19.
62. J. Fletcher, 'Four Indicators of Humanhood—The Enquiry Matures', *The Hastings Center Report* 4 (1975), 4–7.
63. Ibid., 6.
64. R. Veatch, 'Whole-Brain, Neocortical and Higher Brain Related Concepts', in *Death: Beyond Whole-Brain Criteria*, op. cit.
65. D. Wikler, 'Death, Not Dying? Ethical Categories and Persistent Vegetative States', *The Hastings Center Report* 18.1 (1988), 41–7.
66. Upper-brain activity is the currently accepted criterion for the loss of consciousness. However, as with the brainstem criterion, this may change over time should it be discovered that only a certain level or type of upper-brain activity is necessary and sufficient for consciousness or should artificial replacements become possible.
67. R. Veatch, *A Theory of Medical Ethics* (New York: Basic Books, 1981), 242.

68. Ibid., 242–5.
69. Robert Wennberg, op. cit., 159–62.
70. Hans Jonas, 'Against the Stream: Comments on the Definition and Redefinition of Death', in *Ethical Issues in Death and Dying*, Edited by Tom Beauchamp and Seymour Perlin (Englewood Cliffs, NJ: Prentice-Hall, 1978), 51ff.
71. Jocelyn Downie, 'Brain Death and Brain Life', *Bioethics*, vol. 4, no. 3 (1990), 225.
72. Charles Culver and Bernard Gert, op. cit., 182.
73. Edward Bartlett and Stuart Youngner, op. cit., 211.
74. John Stanley, 'More fiddling with the definition of death?' *Journal of Medical Ethics* vol. 13. no. 1. March 1987, 21.
75. Bernard Häring, *Medical Ethics* (Middlegreen, Slough: St Paul Publications, 1974), 132–3.
76. George Lobo, *Moral and Pastoral Questions* (Anand, India: Gujarat Sahitya Prakash, 1985), 248–56.
77. J. Drane, op. cit., 95.
78. A. Flew, in *Euthanasia and the Right to Death*. Edited by A. B. Downing (London: 1974), 33.
79. D. Brock, 'Death and Dying,' in *Medical Ethics*. Edited by R. Veatch (Boston: Jones and Bartlett, 1989), 347–8.
80. P. Singer, *Practical Ethics*, op. cit., 194–5.
81. D. Brock, *Life and Death*, op. cit., 205–7.
82. J. Rachels, 'Active and Passive Euthanasia', *New England Journal of Medicine* 292 (9 January 1975), 78–80.
83. R. Wennberg, *Terminal Choices*, op. cit., 178–9.
84. P. Singer, op. cit., 184.
85. The numbers of patients in a persistent vegetative state and the duration of these states is reported in 'USA: Right to Live, or Right to Die?' *The Lancet*, vol. 337 (12 January 1991).
86. P. Singer, op. cit., 192.
87. The following is a form prepared by the Voluntary Euthanasia Society of England.

To my family and my physician

This Declaration is made by me...........................at a time when I am of sound mind and after careful consideration.

If I am unable to take part in decisions about my medical care owing to my physical or mental incapacity and if I develop one or more of the medical conditions listed in Item Three below and two independent physicians conclude that there is no prospect of my recovery, I declare that my wishes are as follows:

1. I request that my life shall not be sustained by artificial means such as life support system, intravenous fluids or drugs, or by tube feeding.

2. I request that distressing symptoms caused either by the illness or by the lack of food or fluid should be controlled by appropriate sedative treatment, even though such treatment may shorten my life.

3. The said medical conditions are:

(1) Severe and lasting brain damage sustained as a result of injury, including stroke, or disease.

(2) Advanced disseminated malignant disease.

(3) Advanced degenerative disease of the nervous and/or muscular systems with severe limitations of independent mobility, and no satisfactory response to treatment.

(4) Senile or pre-senile dementia e.g. Alzheimer or multi-infarct type.

(5) Other condition of comparable gravity.

* Cross out and initial any condition you do not wish to include.

I further declare that I hereby absolve my medical attendants from any civil liability arising from action taken in response to and in terms of this Declaration.

I reserve my right to revoke this Declaration at any time.

(Signed in the Presence of two witnesses)

Medical emergency card—to be carried on the person
My full name is
Please contact
1. My blood group is
2. Medical information
3. If there is no reasonable prospect of recovery I do NOT wish to be resuscitated or my life to be artificially prolonged. (tick)
4. After death my organs may be used for medical purposes. (tick)

Signature.   *Date*

Refer Ludwig Kennedy, *Euthanasia* (London: Chatto and Windus, 1990), 47–9.

88. Ian Kennedy, (Chair) Working Party of Age Concern England and the Centre of Medical Law and Ethics of King's College London, *The Living Will: Consent to Treatment at the End of Life* (London: Edward Arnold, 1988).

89. Ibid., 29.
90. J. Finnis, '"Living Will" Legislation', in *Euthanasia, Clinical Practice and the Law*. Edited by L. Gormally (London: Linacre Centre for Health Care Ethics, 1994), 167–8.
91. J. Stone, 'Advanced Directives, Autonomy and Unintended Death', *Bioethics* vol. 8, no. 3 (1994), 223.
92. J. Keown, 'The Law and Practice of Euthanasia in The Netherlands', *Law Quarterly Review* 108 (1992), 51–5.
93. Ibid., 57–60.
94. P. Admiraal, 'Justifiable Active Euthanasia in the Netherlands', in *Euthanasia: The Moral Issues*. Edited by R. Baird and S. Rosenbaum (New York: Prometheus Books, 1989), 125.
95. Ibid., 126–7.
96. J. Drane, op. cit., 84.
97. R. Dworkin, *Life's Dominion* (London: HarperCollins, 1993), 181.
98. *Medische beslissingen ron het levenseinde. Het onderzoek voor de commissie onderzoek medische praktijk inzake euthanasie* ('s–Gravenhage: Sdu Uitgeverij Plantijnstraat, 1991). An English translation has been published as P. J. van der Maas et al, *Euthanasia and other Medical Decision at the End of Life* (Elsevier, 1992) (Hereafter van der Maas).
99. P. J. van der Maas, op. cit., 49.
100. C. Gomez, *Regulating Death: Euthanasia and the Case of the Netherlands* (New York: The Free Press, 1991). See also, C. Gomez, 'Euthanasia: Consider the Dutch', in *Mercy or Murder: Euthanasia, Morality & Public Policy*. Edited by K. Overberg (Kansas City: Sheed and Ward, 1993), 161.
101. See 'Dutch doctors support life termination in dementia', *British Medical Journal* 306 (1993), 1364.
102. C. Ciesielski-Carlucci and G. Kimsma, 'The Impact of reporting Cases of Euthanasia in Holland: A Patient and Family Perspective', *Bioethics* vol. 8, no. 2 (1994), 151–8.
103. T. Sheldon, 'The Doctor who Prescribed Suicide', *The Independent*, 30 June 1994, 25.
104. *Gaudium et Spes*, para 27. In *Vatican Council II*, 1981 edition. Edited by A. Flannery (Dublin: Dominican Publications, 1980), 928.
105. 'Every form of direct euthanasia, that is to say, the administration of a narcotic in order to procure or to hasten death, is immoral because it is a claim to dispose directly of life . . . One lays claim to a right of direct disposition whenever one wills the shortening of life as an end or as a means.' Pope Pius XII, Address of 24

NOTES TO PAGES 211–216   285

February 1957 to doctors and surgeons in response to questions by
anaesthetists, AAS 49 (1957), 129–47. See likewise Congregation
for the Doctrine of the Faith, *Iura et Bona* (*Declaration on
Euthanasia*), AAS 72 (1980), 542–52.

106. Pope Pius XII, Address of 24 November 1957, AAS 49 (1957),
     1027–33. Quoted extracts at 1030–32.
107. Congregation for the Doctrine of the Faith, *Declaration on
     Euthanasia,* 1980, no. 17. *In Vatican Council II,* vol. 2. Edited by
     A. Flannery (Dublin: Dominican Publications, 1982), 512.
108. *Declaration on Euthanasia,* op. cit., 511.
109. *Declaration on Euthanasia,* op. cit., 513.
110. *Declaration on Euthanasia,* op. cit., 513–15.
111. *Catechism of the Catholic Church* (Dublin: Veritas, 1994), 491.
112. Pope John Paul II, *Evangelium Vitae* (Vatican City: Libreria
     Editrice Vaticana, 1995), no. 65, 117.
113. Ibid., no. 65, 119. See Second Vatican Ecumenical Council,
     Dogmatic Constitution on the Church, *Lumen Gentium,* no. 25.
114. Ibid., no. 65, 118.
115. *Gaudium et Spes,* no. 24. In *Vatican Council II,* op. cit., 925.
116. Pope John Paul II, Address to Midwives, 26 January 1980; *Acta
     Apostolicae Sedis* 72 (1980), 84–8.
117. A Working Party Report of the Linacre Centre, 'Euthanasia and
     Clinical Practice: Trends, Principles and Alternatives (1982)', in
     Euthanasia, Clinical Practice and the Law. Edited by L. Gormally
     (London: The Linacre Centre for Health Care Ethics, 1994), 51.
118. P. Sporken, *Menschlich sterben* (Dusseldorf: Patmos, 1973), 36ff.
     'As far as I can assess, it seems to me that it can indeed be morally
     justified to shorten this last phase of the dying process drastically
     through active intervention.' 36. See also C. Curran, *Ongoing
     Revision* (Notre Dame, Ind: Fides Publications, 1975), 160. Also
     D. Maguire, *Death by Choice* (Garden City, New York: Image
     Books, 1984), 134, 186.
119. L. Sowle Cahill, 'Respecting Life and Causing Death in the
     Medical Context', *Concilium* 179 (3/1985), 37. See also H.
     Kramer, 'Aktive Euthanasie—christlick?', *Stimmen der Zeit* 203
     (1985), 678; and V. Eid (ed), *Euthanasie onder Soll man auf
     Verlanfen Toten* 1, c. ii.
120. A Working Party Report of the Linacre Centre, op. cit., 53.
121. R. McCormick, 'The New Medicine and Morality', *Theology
     Digest* 21 (1973), 315–20.
122. A. Holderegger, *Il suicidio* (Assisi: Cittadella, 1979), 367–9,
     435ff.
123. H. Rotter, *Die Wurde des Lebens* (Innsbruck: Tyrolia, 1987), 117.

124. K. Kelly, 'Why Should Catholics Oppose Euthanasia Legislation?' *Catholic Gazette* (April 1970), 5–6.

125. In a very convincing way that fact has been evidenced by the alternative of the St Christopher Hospice, founded by Dr Cecily Saunders for terminally ill patients. In these hospices no artificial prolongation of life is undertaken, not even intravenous feeding. Its formula is a blend of pain relief, tender care and the close involvement of the family in the process of dying. 40,000 Britons who die each year of cancer are treated in a hospice or receive hospice-style care at home. The average life-span of a patient in hospice treatment is just three weeks. The cost is sizeable, £350 a day. But this is no more than in the intensive care facilities, where most hospice patients would otherwise end up. Euthanasia is not practised by the hospice.

126. K. Kelly, 'Why Should Catholics Oppose Euthanasia Legislation?', op. cit., 5–6.

127. A. Holderegger, op. cit., 436.

128. Dr Helene Dupuis, Professor of Bioethics at Leiden University in the Netherlands, is convinced 'that no lung-cancer patient in this country dies of natural causes' (*Newsweek*, 14 May 1988, 47).

129. *Declaration on Euthanasia*, op. cit., 513.

130. P. Verspieren, op. cit., 108 f.

131. P. Admiraal, op. cit., 84.

132. L. Sowle Cahill, 'Respecting Life and Causing Death in the Medical Context', *Concilium* 179 (1985), 37.

133. B. Häring, *Free and Faith in Christ*, vol. 3 (London: St Pauls Publications, 1981), 88.

134. Board for Social Responsibility of the Church of England, *On Dying Well* (Church Information Office, Church House, Dean's Yard, 1975), 1–67.

135. Ibid., 7–9.

136. J. S. Habgood, 'Euthanasia—A Christian View', *Journal of the Royal Society of Health* 3 (1974), 124, 126.

137. *On Dying Well*, op. cit., 12.

138. Ibid., 21.

139. Ibid., 22.

140. R. McCormick, 'Care for the Dying and Euthanasia', in *Notes on Moral Theology 1965–through 1980* (London: University Press of America, 1981), 602–5.

141. House of Bishops, *Euthanasia: A Statement by the House of Bishops*, Press release, 29 October 1992.

142. Report of the Board of Social responsibility of the Church of

Scotland, *Euthanasia* (Edinburgh: The Church of Scotland Board of Social Responsibility, 1994), 7.
143. Ibid., 8.
144. Ibid., 26.
145. Methodist Conference, *A Methodist Statement on Euthanasia*, 1974, nos. 16–24.
146. 'Euthanasia and the Law', *Briefing* 22 July 1993. Refer *Doctrine and Life* 43 (1993), 493.
147. Ibid., 496.
148. Ibid., 494.
149. *Declaration on Euthanasia*, op. cit., 514–16.
150. A. Moraczewski, 'Euthanasia in the Light of a Contemporary Theology of Death', in *Euthanasia Symposium* (proceedings of a symposium sponsored by the Catholic Hospital Conference of Saskatchewan, Alberta, and British Columbia, 3–4 October 1974), 19–38.
151. C. Curran, *Politics, Medicine and Christian Ethics* (Philadelphia, 1973), 161–2.
152. P. Ramsey, *The Patient is a Person* (New Haven: Yale University Press, 1970), 157–60.
153. R. McCormick, 'Notes on Moral Theology', *Theological Studies* 34 (1973), 167.
154. J. Fletcher, 'Sanctity of Life versus Quality of Life', in *Euthanasia: The Moral Issues*. Edited by R. Baird and S. Rosenbaum (New York: Prometheus Books, 1989), 69.
155. J. Rachels, 'Active and Passive Euthanasia', in *Euthanasia: The Moral Issues*, op. cit., 48–9.
156. J. Rachels, 'Active and Passive Euthanasia', in *Mercy or Murder*. Edited by K. Overberg (Kansas City: Sheed & Ward, 1993), 23–32. This essay first appeared in *New England Journal of Medicine* 292 (1975), 78–80.
157. Ibid., 30.
158. P. Singer, 'Philosophers Are Back on the Job', *New York Times Magazine*, 7 July 1974, 6 ff.
159. Document *Dans le cadre*, 'Quelques questions d'ethique relatives aux grands malades et aux mourants', of 27 June 1981, sections 3.1f. Cited by K. Peschke, 'The Pros and Cons of Euthanasia Re-examined', *The Irish Theological Quarterly* 58 (1992), 15.
160. Notably Paul Ramsey in *The Patient as Person*. Ramsey's understanding in turn derived from his reading of Gerald Kelly, 'The Duty of Using Artificial Means of Preserving Life', *Theological Studies* 11 (1950), 203–20, and the same author's

'The Duty to Preserve Life' *Theological Studies* 12 (1951), 550–56.

161. Pope Pius XII, AAS 39 (1957), 1027–33.
162. P. Ramsey, op. cit., 122.
163. To avoid ambiguities some writers suggest the terminology should be abandoned. E.g. Paul Ramsey *Ethics at the Edges of Life. Medical and Legal Intersections* 1978, 155; Robert Veatch, *Death, Dying and the Biological Revolution* 1976, 110.
164. W. Frankena, *Ethics* (Englewood Cliffs, NJ: 1973), 42.
165. S. Bok, 'Death and Dying: Ethical Views', in *Encyclopedia of Bioethics* I, 27.
166. Refer D. McCarthy, and E. Bayer, *Handbook on Critical Life Issues* (Braintree, Mass: Pope John Center, 1988), 151.
167. G. Kelly, *Medico-Moral Problems* (St Louis, MO: The Catholic Hospital Association, 1957), 129.
168. D. McCarthy and E. Bayer, op. cit., 152–3.
169. *Declaration on Euthanasia*, 515.
170. For example, Paul Ramsey, *Patient as Person* (New Haven: Yale University Press, 1970); and *Dying*, Considerations concerning the passage from life to death, Task Force on Human Life, Anglican Church of Canada, edited by L. Whytehed and P. Chedwick (Toronto, Can.: The Anglican Book Centre, 1980).
171. J. Fletcher, 'Sanctity of Life versus Quality of Life', op. cit., 86.
172. B. Häring, op. cit., 102.
173. R. McCormick, 'To Save or Let Die', in *Quality of Life: The New Medical Dilemma*. Edited by J. Walter and T. Shannon (New York, Paulist Press, 1990), 31.
174. R. McCormick, op. cit., 32.
175. James Walter, 'The Meaning and Validity of Quality of Life Judgments in Contemporary Roman Catholic Medical Ethics', in *Quality of Life*, op. cit., 80.
176. Editorial, 'A New Ethic for Medicine and Society', *California Medicine*, September 1970, 67–8.
177. Leonard Weber, *Who Shall Live?* (New York: Paulist Press, 1976), 41–2.
178. For example, see W. Reich, 'Quality of Life and Defective Newborn Children: An Ethical Analysis', in *Decision Making and the Defective Newborn: Proceedings of a Conference on Spina Bifida and Ethics*. Edited by C. Swinyard (Springfield, IL: Charles Thomas, 1978), 489–511; and B. Johnstone, 'The Sanctity of Life, the Quality of Life and the New "Baby Doe" Law', *Linacre Quarterly* 52 (1985), 258–70.
179. B. Johnstone, 'The Sanctity of Life', op. cit., 263.

180. W. Reich, 'Quality of Life and Defective Newborn Children', op. cit., 504.
181. J. Walter, op. cit., 84.
182. Ibid., 85–6.
183. J. Lynn, and J. Childress, 'Must Patients Always Be Given Food and Water?' *Hastings Center Report* 13 (1983), 17–21.
184. D. Brock, 'Death and Dying', op. cit., 353.
185. M. Siegler and A. Weisbard, 'Against the Emerging Stream', *Arch Intern Med* 145 (1985), 129–31.
186. D. Brock, 'Death and Dying', op. cit., 354.
187. Oregon and Washington Bishops, 'Living and Dying Well', *Origins* 21 (1991), 346–52. See also Oregon and Washington Bishops, 'Living and Dying Well', in *Mercy and Murder*. Edited by K. Overberg (Kansas City: Sheed and Ward, 1993), 183–202.
188. Oregon and Washington Bishops, op. cit., 349–50.
189. Ibid., 350. Additional support for the Washington and Oregon Bishops' Statement on the moral option to withhold or withdraw nutrition and fluids from dying patients or those in a persistent vegetative condition are found in the Texas Bishops' Statement 'On Withdrawing Artificial Nutrition and Hydration', *Origins* 21 (1990), 53ff; United States Bishops' Committee for Pro-Life Activities, 'The Rights of the Terminally Ill', *Origins* 16 (1987), 222–6; Catholic Health Association of Wisconsin, 'Guidelines on the Use of Nutrition and Fluids on Catholic Health Care Facilities', (1989); R. McCormick, 'Nutrition-Hydration: The New Euthanasia?' in *The Critical Calling* (Washington, DC: Georgetown University Press, 1989); J. Paris, 'The Catholic Tradition on the Use of Nutrition and Fluids', in *Birth, Suffering and Death*. Edited by K. Wildes (Dordrecht: Kluwer, 1991). See also Lisa Sowle Cahill's coverage of the issue in *Theological Studies* 52 (1991), 110–19.
190. The Massachusetts Catholic Conference, *The Health Care Proxy Bill: A Catholic Guide* (Boston: Pilot Publishing Co., 1 December 1990), 1–8, at 3.
191. Cited by R. McCormick, op. cit., 255–6.
192. R. McCormick, '"Moral Considerations" Ill Considered', in *Mercy or Murder,* op. cit., 252.
193. The American Medical Association, the American Academy of Neurology.
194. D. Brodeur *Health Progress*, June 1985. Cited in R. McCormick, op. cit., 256.
195. K. O'Rourke, cited by R. McCormick, op. cit., 258–9.

196. K. O'Rourke, *America*, 22 November 1986, cited by K. Kelly, *The Tablet*, 13 March 1993, 333.

197. R. McCormick, op. cit., 259.

198. L. Schneiderman, N. Jecker and A. Jonsen, *Annals of Internal Medicine*, 15 June 1990, Cited by R. McCormick, op. cit., 260.

199. The proposed conduct has the aim . . . of terminating the life of Anthony Bland; . . . the conduct . . . is intended to be the cause of death (Lord Mustil at 35,4 4); the whole purpose of stopping artificial feeding is to bring about the death of Anthony Bland (Lord Browne-Wilkinson at 28); the intention to bring about the patient's death is there (Lord Lowry at 23).

200. *Briefing*, 12 August 1993. Reproduced in *Doctrine and Life* 43 (1993), 492–3.

201. Bishop Budd of Plymouth said that feeding Tony Bland is the kind of basic care owed to every human being, not a form of 'extraordinary care' which might properly be withheld (*The Tablet*, 28 November 1992). Many American bishops have repeatedly made similar statements. See also: Pontifical Academy of Sciences, *The Artificial Prolongation of Life and the Exact Definition of the Moment of Death*, 30 October 1985; Committee for Pro-Life Activities in the US National Conference of Catholic Bishops, *Guidelines for Legislation on Life-Sustaining Treatment*, 10 November 1984, and *Statement on Uniform Rights of the Terminally Ill* Act, June 1986; New Jersey Catholic Conference, *Amicus curiae brief in the Matter of Nancy Ellen Jobes*, October 1986.

202. Those regarding tube-feeding as a medical treatment which can properly be withdrawn from the permanently comatose include: J. Paris & R. McCormick, 'The Catholic tradition on the use of nutrition and fluids', *America*, 2 May 1987, 358; R. McCormick, 'Caring or starving? The Case of Claire Conroy', *America*, 6 April 1986; E. Bayer, 'Is food always obligatory?' *Ethics and Medicine*, 10 (1985); K. O'Rourke, 'The AMA Statement on tube feeding: an ethical analysis', *America*, 22 November 1986, 321–3, 331; D. Callahan, 'On feeding the dying', *Hastings Center Report*, 131(5) (October 1983).

   Those regarding tube-feeding as a medical treatment or quasi-medical treatment, but one which should normally be maintained for the comatose include: J. Connery, 'In the matter of Claire Conroy', *Linacre Quarterly* 52 (1985), 321–34 and 'The ethics of withholding/withdrawing nutrition and hydration', *Linacre Quarterly* 54 (1987); W. May, 'Feeding and hydrating the permanently unconscious and other vulnerable persons', *Issues* in *Law and Medicine* 3 (1987), 203–17 and 'Statement in support of the New Jersey Catholic Conference', in R. Barry, *Medical Ethics: Essays on Abortion and Euthanasia* (New York: Peter Lang, 1989), 263–72; G. Grisez, 'Should nutrition and hydration be provided to permanently unconscious and other mentally disabled persons?' *Linacre Quarterly* 57 (1990), 30–43.

Those opposed to regarding tube-feeding as a medical treatment, who argue instead that it is part of the normal or minimum care due to all patients, include: R. Barry, 'Facing hard cases: the ethics of assisted feeding', *Issues in Law and Medicine*, 2 (1986), 100–106, and 'The ethics of providing life-sustaining nutrition and fluids to incompetent patients', *Journal of Family & Culture*, 1 (2); J. Piccione, 'The tradition of care', *Euthanasia Review*, 1 (2), 129–31; W. Smith, 'Judaeo-Christian teaching on euthanasia: definitions, distinctions and decisions', *Linacre Quarterly* 54 (1987).

203. A. Fisher, 'On Not Starving the Unconscious', *New Blackfriars* 74 (1993), 133–5.
204. Gerald Kelly published *Medico-Moral Problems* in 1960 and Edwin Healy published *Medical Ethics* in 1956.
205. K. Kelly, *The Tablet*, 13 March 1993, 333.
206. Ibid., 333.
207. D. Brock, 'Death and Dying', op. cit., 355.

INDEX

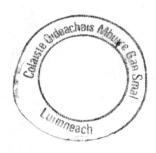

Religion e Morality (241 BKW 1044S)

" " 200-9 (BRN 2472)

2

241 0

230 · 01

370 114.

150 · 1952